To Helyn —
may the angels
hover near

Love

Charlie Shedd

Remember, I Love You

Other Books by Charlie W. Shedd

On Marriage

Letters to Karen
Letters to Philip
Talk to Me
Celebration in the Bedroom
How to Stay in Love
Bible Study Together: Making Marriage Last
Praying Together: Making Marriage Last

For Young People

The Stork Is Dead
You Are Somebody Special (edited by Charlie Shedd)
Is Your Family Turned On?

For Parents and Grandparents

You Can Be a Great Parent
Smart Dads I Know
The Best Dad Is a Good Lover
A Dad Is for Spending Time With
Grandparents: Then God Created Grandparents
Grandparents: Family Book
Tell Me a Story: Stories for Grandchildren

To Help You Manage Your Life

Time for All Things
The Fat Is in Your Head
Devotions for Dieters
Pray Your Weight Away
Getting Through to the Wonderful You

Ideas for Churches

The Exciting Church: Where People Really Pray
The Exciting Church: Where They Give Their Money Away
The Exciting Church: Where They Really Use the Bible
The Pastoral Ministry of Church Officers
How to Develop a Tithing Church
How to Develop a Praying Church

On Writing

If I Can Write, You Can Write

Remember, I Love You
Martha's Story

Charlie W. Shedd

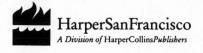

HarperSanFrancisco
A Division of HarperCollins*Publishers*

FIRST EDITION

Library of Congress Cataloging-in-Publication Data

Shedd, Charlie W.
    Remember, I love you : Martha's story / Charlie W. Shedd.—1st ed.
        p. cm.
    ISBN 0-06-067256-0
    1. Shedd, Martha. 2. Shedd, Charlie W. 3. Christian
biography—United States. 4. Married people—Religious
life. 5. Cancer—Patients—United States—Biography. I. Title.
BR1725.S452S44   1990
209'.2—dc20   90-37715
[B]   CIP

90 91 92 93 94 HAD 10 9 8 7 6 5 4 3 2 1

This edition is printed on acid-free paper that meets the American National Standards Institute Z39.48 Standard.

Contents

PASTOR'S WIFE
59

TOGETHER
89

MALIGNANT
121

BROKEN PIECES
157

DEDICATION
171

Acknowledgments

To Roland Seboldt, acquisitions editor of Harper & Row.
   He came to me at a time
      when I was shattered, scattered
        and certain I could never write again.
   He assured me, inspired me
      and brought the gift of renewed hope.
                 Thank you, Roland.

To Diane, Methodist minister, Martha's good friend, and
mine.
   She took my jumbled notes,
      my scribbled scraps of recall and memoirs.
   From countless pages, from bits and pieces,
      she fashioned an outline.
   Editor extraordinary, friend extraordinary,
      happy surprise.
                 Thank you, Diane.

To Ione, super secretary.
   She did and re-did
      every draft of the manuscript
        on Martha's computer.
   Skillful, patient, fun lady.
                 Thank you, Ione.

To Martha Sprugel Thompson and Margie Johnson Kelting,
  Stars of that exciting basketball team.
    By many phone calls and visits
      plus data from scrapbooks and diaries,
    We recreated the thrilling story
      of success when no one expected it.
               Thank you, Martha T. and Margie K.

To Jacques, Paula, Treva Jane, Bonnie, and Melanie,
  Readers of the first and second drafts.
    For clarification, for reaction,
      but above all for making Martha's special love come
      through
      as we had all experienced it.
               Thank you, dear friends.

Then to Karen, my lawyer daughter.
  She evaluated the final manuscript
    to blend the words with her mother's character.
  Sharpening, honing, cutting, polishing,
    she applied the final touches.
               Thank you, Karen.

And, finally, to all those men and women of the Lord,
  who have lived with Him
    so long, so well
      that they are really speaking for Him
        when they say,
          "Remember, I love you."

Charlie Shedd
Athens, Georgia
1990

Prologue

"Remember, I love you."

This was the Martha blessing, and with special tones for special times she said it.

In her mellow voice, it was almost uncanny the many ways she made it sound:

Reassuring, for the down days—encouraging

Healing, for hurts of heart—mending

Calm, for moments of tension—cooling

Then again, the very opposite of cool—warm,
    exciting, inviting.

Never overused, though, it was prompted as if from some sensitive timer in her soul.

She said it to those with whom she agreed and to those with whom she disagreed. She said it to her children and to all children. To the teenagers she taught, to those with whom she counseled. Couples newly married and couples struggling in their middle years, singles and those single again, empty-nesters and the elderly. To all these she said it.

But especially she said it to me. For me, she even had a certain smile that, without a single sound, would say without a single doubt, "Remember, I love you."

EARLY LOVE

Deep calleth unto deep.
Psalm 42:7, KJV

The Song with My Name

Her voice was like a song, and considering her subject, that was surprising. She was reading history. "Important dates," the teacher said. Important people too, plus places important. But why should *I* care?

The little community where I grew up had several things going for it, none better than the school possibilities for eighth graders. We could choose any one of four high schools. We were an unincorporated village with no educational loyalty. So which would it be: East Waterloo, West Waterloo, Cedar Falls, or Teacher's College High?

For those of us on the eighth-grade football team there was no debate. Every year West Waterloo finished strong, often winning the state championship. Every year their best made all-state. Some would be offered scholarships to Big Ten schools. A few in West High's history had even gone to the pros.

Recruiting is nothing new. Coaches from the four high schools would scout our games. If they liked what they saw, they'd visit in our home, meet our parents, give us the pitch. "Come play for us. Can't miss. You'll go a long way." Interpreted by junior high fantasy, that meant way, way up to the

Bears (our nearest pro team was Chicago). Heady stuff for an eighth-grader.

In early June the town of Cedar Falls annexed our little village. There went my choices. I was to enroll in the nearest school, and that meant Cedar Falls High. Their last winning season? Could anyone remember?

What do we do when fate intervenes and our hopes tumble? Despair in junior high may not be worse than despair at any other age. Perhaps it only *seems* worse. For me, this was the lowest blow of all the world's low blows that summer.

So off I went to Cedar Falls High at a slow shuffle, pouting all the way.

Huge question on the eighth-grade level: "Why would God do me this way? Me! Future all-stater, all-American, all-pro, all-done-in-with-despair. How *could* He?"

The first day in history class I had my answer: the song with my name!

Football season opened Friday night. We'd been practicing for three weeks. Before school started, the coach had been shaping us up. Now I was looking out the classroom window, wondering, will I be in the starting lineup? Freshmen usually served some bench time, but I did have a chance. We needed bulk in the line, and I was bulky.

Then I heard the voice again, and I turned to look at her. She was wearing a big yellow sweater, yellow skirt. There was an aura about her I'd never seen before, a new sound too. What was this in all that data she was reading? A song? A song with my name: "Charlie. Charlie. Charlie." But it was more than that; this was like some kind of personal Pentecost ("Suddenly there came a sound from heaven," Acts 2).

We were in several classes together, and as I studied her, I picked up an interesting ritual. Always before the class-come-to-order-now bell she would go to the teacher's desk and sharpen her pencil. I liked that. Be prepared, and especially be sharp.

Not being skilled in the ways of first love, I pondered an approach. And how was this for an amateur? At home I scrounged for dull pencils, and every day I joined her at the pencil sharpener.

Initially these meetings were somewhat awkward, but before long we were conversing. At the start there was only a trickle of words, because she was shy. But since I wasn't, we were soon into a rather nice pattern of teen communication.

Then we found our theme. She liked to ice skate, and so did I. Most Iowa teens in our day skated. We skated well because we skated often, and we skated for many reasons. Reason one for some of us? Boys and girls together.

Almost every weekend she and I would meet at Washington Pond. Her parents knew she'd be all right there with her many cousins, mostly girls. Mothers and fathers sometimes miss the full picture. Hers did. They knew absolutely nothing about her newfound interest—me! Naturally her cousins knew, and they were excited.

All of us loved Washington Pond. We loved it for a meeting place, and we loved what happened there. We also loved the setting: big pond, lots of ice, beautiful overhanging trees, and a huge bonfire to warm ourselves. There were also miscellaneous coves for those who warmed better with a touch of privacy.

The way of a man with a maid on ice is something special. Flow. Rhythm, swing, and sway. Share some sweet talk, and hold me close so I won't stumble.

Those of us who knew the pond knew also the narrow outlets leading to the river. When the ice was at its best, up the river we'd go to our favorite bower. We'd brush the snow from a fallen log and cozy down for a real visit. "See the sunlight on these icicles, see the limbs bending low? Perfect, isn't it?" And it was. For tender young love like ours, absolutely perfect.

When summer came, there were canoes at the marina. Some of these belonged to friends who never used them. I also had a rowboat—solid, well built. I should know; I built it. I also built it nonsubmergible. "A+" my shop teacher gave me, and that was impressive. So was the yellow I painted my boat.

Yellow was her favorite color, and I was her favorite fellow, and this was her favorite river. So off we would go to our favorite cove, where even the birds were singing our favorite song.

How could a friendship born in winters like that and summers so idyllic be for anything else than a love divinely touched? Was all this the reason behind that unwelcome annexation closing down my high-school choices?

I think it was.

No Big Ten football for me, nor all-American. No pick of the pro teams either. But out of the broken pieces of that dream there she came: *Martha! All—everything for me!*

You can pour love's soft assurances
Into my ear for hours,
And I will only thirst for more:
As long as you can speak,
I'll long to hear you speak of love.

"I Think You're Wonderful"

Bulky I was, but that's not all. From growing too fast I was awkward. From eating too much I was loaded down with pounds too many. I was also loaded down with inner confusion. Big on the outside, inside my self-image was a real pygmy. "You're a bad one. Strictly no good."

How I accumulated all these negatives is not for this book. How I came out of them is, and her name was Martha.

Shy she was, but not when it came to affirming her new-found friend. As I began sharing my poverty-stricken opinion of me, she'd take my hand. Then, looking at me with eyes expressing something I had never seen before, she would say, "Charlie, I think you're wonderful. If you're so bad, how come you're on the football team already? Why did we elect you homeroom president? You're fun, that's why. Don't you know how many friends you have? I'm not going to let you think you're bad. *I* like you, and *I* think you're wonderful!"

Most early teens are concentrating on the downs of life. How could I be so lucky? Here she was, my ego builder supreme, herald of the positives. How did she get this way?

The Danish Lutheran church of our early years was noted for its serious training: grueling confirmation, on and on, week after week, month after month, one year, two. Catechism, memory work, most of it mired in dismal theology.

Over and over, Martha said, she heard over and over again Martin Luther's main theme: "The purpose of our Christian life is to resist the devil." Martha's class had even been given "the list." Another list to learn, the list of all the devil's bad little devils out to get good boys and girls.

But what if there weren't all these devils little and big in your particular life? What if your mother majored in the joy of the Lord? What if your father loved you? What if your little brother was more pal than pest? What if there were all those fun cousins to enjoy?

Surrounded as she was by good, for her there had to be something better than all this focus on evil. Could it be that her old-country pastor was wrong?

The Danish Lutherans have a built-in reverence for all clergy. Martha had been brought up with this: "Pastor says it. You believe it!" But now coming out from the back of her thoughts was a lurking question, "Could this poor man have a damaged picture of God as He really is?"

She decided the pastor *did* have a problem. From here on she would respect the good in him, but she would reject altogether some of his teaching. Especially she would reject the lesson he taught about her baby cousins.

Some years before, Aunt Camilla had given birth to twins. It was evident they wouldn't live, so the pastor was called to baptize them. One, still breathing, received the sacrament. For the other it was too late. The baptized baby, he said, went to heaven; the unbaptized didn't.

Every year in confirmation and in church school, Martha heard this same legalistic emphasis, this same illustration. But finally, she heard it once too often and made her decision. From now on she would not be her pastor's kind of Lutheran, or Martin Luther's either. She would respect the good in her church's teaching, but enough was enough.

The God she knew cared about all babies, baptized and unbaptized. Even before they were born, her God treated them all alike because He loved them all alike, no exception!

———

So wouldn't the God who made little babies and loved what He made do this too? Wouldn't He maybe take an optimistic view of the potential in her teenage boyfriend? Of course He would, no maybe about it.

Doesn't the Bible say before it is two chapters old, "Then God looked over everything He had made, and behold it was excellent in every way"? So what if things weren't exactly as He'd created them? Didn't this same God have the power to restore? He could make His original excellent again. Wonderful.

Basic theology—nothing casual, nothing fake—four redeeming words to one needy teenager: "I think you're wonderful."

Over the years she would discover where I wasn't wonderful. But that also was part of her theology. She had been taught—and she believed it—"All have sinned and come short of the glory of God." Yet always, for her, what mattered most was the glory of God behind the sin.

I, too, had been brought up with heavy theology. My brand was John Calvin. A brilliant theologian. Two of his

melancholy drumbeats were "original sin" and "total deprav-
ity." In the version I was getting, Calvin was dreadfully
lacking in mercy, grace, love, and encouragement. To me, his
theme came off this way: "You are bad because you were born
bad." (Interesting note: One of his biographers says John Calvin had kidney stones, regularly. I had one once, and I can
guarantee that anyone cursed with kidney stones regularly
could not be optimistic about anything!)

Is it any wonder that I fell deeply in love with this teenage
theologian who told me until I believed it:

"The real you is not bad, Charlie!
In the beginning God made you good!
And looking through to His original,
I think you're wonderful."

Ye shall go out with joy . . . the
mountains and the hills shall break forth
before you into singing, and all the trees
of the field shall clap their hands.

Isaiah 55:12, KJV

———————

"You Be Good to Marta! Ja?"

Marius was a wide man and very strong. He had been
made that way by working on a Danish horse farm. He was
only eleven when he and his brothers left home to escape a new
stepmother.

Hard to believe? Not by conditions in Denmark almost a
hundred years ago. Child labor laws, nil. The rule was, "If
they're strong enough, they're old enough." So, naturally
hearty at eleven, he was hired for the horse farm. Now he
would become even stronger. He could harness and haul, plow
and harrow, plant, put up hay, water and feed. And, said he,
"I was the nightwatchman. I slept in the manger." (That
sounds far out too, doesn't it, but I never knew him to tell a
lie. A firm believer, he knew the Ten Commandments and
tried to live by them.)

With that kind of character, plus a powerful back and
powerful arms, he came to America at twenty-one. He must
have been a premium product in the work market.

Marius was a loving father, very protective of his two
children. His son Herloff, cut from his father's cloth, soon
showed his ability to make his own way. But Martha now, she
would be different. Every father worth the name has special
concerns for his daughter, and so too did Marius.

Because she was beautiful, he must have known someone would be knocking one day. And I was the someone.

======

The first time I came, they let me in. Her brother and I were friends. He had vouched for me Martha said, and vouching I needed. Her parents did not know their daughter and I were already well acquainted. All that ice skating together those winter nights had served us well. Rowing upstream to our cove those summer afternoons was no detriment either. We *were* well acquainted.

Before my first visit, according to Martha, there had been considerable discussion. And she never tired of describing this one smiler:

"His father is a preacher."

"Is he a Lutheran preacher?"

"No. He's a Presbyterian."

"Well he can come once maybe."

Nervous, I rapped on her door. She let me in, parents hovering, waiting for the introduction. Immediate rapport. The minute they saw me, the minute I saw them, the chasm closed, and we were future kin. From that day on it was dinner Sunday noons, popcorn in the evenings, and if the evening went on, another special feature: ten o'clock curfew.

Her parents (I could hardly believe such good fortune) always retired early: nine o'clock. That gave us one hour alone together for strengthening our friendship. Also for tutoring.

Martha was brilliant in math, chemistry, and physics. I wasn't. My specialties were debate, drama, football, and Martha. I wonder how I would have done in science and other trivial subjects without her expert tutoring? But no matter how necessary the tutoring, always, every night, with the first stroke of ten on their somber hall clock came word from the bedroom, "Ten o'clock, Charlie. Good night."

You can believe I went.

———

This was not our only ceremony, man to man. One thing for sure, Marius and I both knew his little girl was extra special. And if I hadn't known, I certainly would have following a second firm reminder.

This one came soon after we began car dating. We were standing together, Marius and I. Here by my questionable Ford convertible he initiated this ritual, a ritual destined to continue over many dates and all the years of our courtship.

Tapping me on the shoulder, he looked me straight in the eye and said, "You be good to Marta. Ja?"

To which I answered, "Ja!"

Marius and I became best friends. We became the kind of friends who could talk about anything, everything, heart to heart. But one thing we never *did* discuss. Not once did he tell me what he meant by "be good," and not once did I ask him for his definition. Not once either did he ask me what I meant by my "ja!"

Through the years I can still feel that firm tap on my shoulder and his deep voice in Danish brogue saying, "You be good to Marta. Ja?"

———

Doesn't every woman need a man who will "be good" to her? Ja!

Doesn't every man need a woman who will "be good" to him? Ja!

And doesn't every man also need a woman to be good to? Ja?

Ja!

"I tell you the truth, I think if there
hadn't been a door in the locker room
we'd have gone through the wall to win
for your Martha."

The Coach Who Said, "I Love You"

When Martha finished college, she was one of the fortunate graduates. For teachers, job openings were way down. In
the late 1930s, all things, including spirits, were down. So
when Martha was hired to teach home economics, we celebrated.

It was a tiny school, tiny town, tiny outlook on nearly
everything, with one exception: hopes for girls' basketball
were big, big.

When Martha arrived on the scene, her principal sum-
moned her for an initial interview. "Miss Petersen," he began,
"you have been selected to coach girls' basketball."

"What? I should coach girls' basketball? Our high school
didn't even play girls' basketball. I've hardly even seen girls'
basketball. You can't mean me."

"Yes, you. The school board won't have a man coaching
girls' basketball. Doesn't look good. So it's you."

"But I came here to teach home economics."

"Sure. We'll let you do that too. But what counts in this
town is basketball, girls' basketball. And here's one thing more.
We've never had a winning season; you better have one." End
of interview!

They had their winning season. Game after game they won, week after week, on the road, at home. Now and then they lost but most of the time it was win, win, win.

Basketball *is* big in Iowa. Especially it's big when little school beats big school. Super story—see them play their hearts out.

How did she do it, this inexperienced coach with inexperienced players? Every Wednesday morning I called her from Chicago (I was in seminary). Saturday morning too, I called. They played Tuesday night and Friday.

Most of the time, good news: "We won."

"How did you do it?"

"I don't know."

"I can't believe you."

"Neither can I."

Then it was on to more important things. And always before we hung up, "Remember, I love you" from her.

"I love you, too," from me.

Still, there was that question, How *did* she do it?

———

Years later I learned the secret. It was Sweetheart Night in an Iowa town, and I was the speaker. Big event, fun occasion, room packed. When it was over, I was at the speaker's table autographing books, shaking hands, saying good night.

Off to the side stood a nice-looking couple, grandparent types, waiting. Waiting for what? Were they folks I should know? Folks with a problem? ("Please, Lord, not that; I'm all done in.") When the hall emptied, here they came.

"Dr. Shedd," she began, "I am Martha Sprugel Thompson." Wasn't this some distant bell ringing in my memory? It was. "You wouldn't remember me," she continued, "but I was on your wife's basketball team the year we won so many games. I thought you might like to know how she coached and the reason we won."

"This," I said, "I can hardly wait to hear."

"Well, the reason we won," she went on, "is because of who she was and what she told us. Whenever we were heading into a big game, or needing points, or playing overtime, or not doing our best, your Martha would gather us around her. Then she would hold out the ball and say, 'Girls, this is the basketball. You know I don't know much about it, but *remember, I love you.*'

"You know, when she came to coach us she was only four years older than we were," Mrs. Thompson mused. (This is a gray-haired grandmother now, recalling events from fifty years ago.) "When she first said she loved us, we couldn't believe what we were hearing. So we tested her. We tried everything, some things not very nice, to see if she meant what she was saying. Then when we knew she *did* mean it, we decided nobody was going to beat us! I tell you the truth, I think if there hadn't been a door in the locker room we'd have gone through the wall to win for your Martha."

===

One morning my telephone rang. It was another member of Martha's basketball team, and her name was Margie Johnson. I remembered this much right away: she and Martha had been especially good friends. To Martha, Margie was extra special. There were many reasons why Margie was special, but this was one for sure.

During the 1930s, dollars were scarce. Families did some unusual things to get by. Example? Suppose there weren't enough quarters for all the family to ride the school bus or buy lunch? Or too few dollars for clothes? Someone had to stay home. Someone had to take the place of a hired hand, put up hay, milk, plant, cultivate. Later, when an older brother or sister graduated, the next fall that someone could go back to school again.

That is what happened to Margie. She had missed the ninth grade. Now she was back, and who should she meet in the hall but Martha.

"I'm the new basketball coach. Why don't you come out for the team? You look like you'd make a good player. I think you'd enjoy it and I'd enjoy you."

Margie came out, and she was exactly what the new coach thought she would be: a good, good player. So good, in fact, she made the honor teams. And when she finished high school, wonder of wonders: Margie, ninth-grade dropout by necessity, country girl from a tiny town, was invited to join a traveling beauty college team from Des Moines. Now she would play big league, playing southern states, eastern states, Canada. Entertaining the fans. Winning, winning, winning.

There is another side to this story I like. Margie *was* someone the new coach enjoyed.

"Your Martha took me to her home in Cedar Falls for a weekend I'll never forget. She took me to her college campus, and I couldn't believe there were buildings so tall. And when she put me on the train for home, I'll never forget this either: she gave me a bracelet. I wore it and wore it and kept it all these years.

"My mother died when I was five, and there were five of us. We missed so many things, so you can imagine the feeling I got when your Martha said, "Remember, I love you."

On the wall of our bedroom hung a picture of Martha and her team. We could see it from our bed, so sometimes we'd reminisce. She'd tell me again how frightened she'd been, coaching and not knowing how. Then she would tell me how she settled down to learn what she could as fast as she could. She read. She studied. She talked with people who knew basketball.

One thing she learned was that if her team scored more points than the other team, there was hardly any way they could lose that game. (I smiled when she first told me that, but this was vintage Martha: get down to the basics—fast.) But even this jewel was not enough. So here came another basic: "To score more than the other team, we must practice more than the other team."

So they practiced. They practiced shooting mostly. Before school, lunch hour, after school, Saturdays, and Sunday afternoons. Practice, practice, practice. Shoot!

"And why would we practice till we were sure our arms would fall off and our legs wouldn't hold us up any longer? We'd practice like that because we knew our coach meant it when she said,

'Remember, I love you.' "

The practice of stillness is cumulative, like
a snowball growing upon itself. It creates
great quiet spaces within.

Glenn Clark

"Shhh!"

"I can still hear her saying, 'Shhh!' She taught us some
things about basketball, but those weren't the most important
lessons. The lesson I treasure most is Martha's emphasis on the
value of quiet."

Straight from where it happened, another member of the
team tells her story. "Most coaches use halftime to ream out
their team or give a pep talk. Do you know what Martha did?
She took us in the home ec room (or maybe a library if we
were the visiting team) and made each of us lie down on a
table. Then she would give a little speech I remember so well:
'Let's not talk about basketball now. Let's have a quiet time.
If we are quiet, strength will come, and wisdom. Don't talk.
Listen. Shhh!'

"She was so right. You simply can't believe the way we
would play together in the second half. Often we had a
rhythm and flow that made us almost unbeatable.

"That quiet time did things for us nothing else could do.
I don't mean just about basketball. I mean about living. That
simple practice has blessed me all my life. And sometimes when
I need it most, I can still hear her saying, 'Shhh!' "

If the quiet time worked so well, why didn't she use that
technique before their games? "Quiet at a time like that?"

Martha mused. "Have you ever been in a small-town cracker-box gymnasium just before game time? Band. Cheerleaders. Screaming crowd. The biggest event in this town's week. Everyone going crazy, including the girls on my team. But at the half, the mood is altogether different—especially if our team is behind. Even if we're winning, the girls are done in. *This* is the time for quiet. Refreshment for body, mind, soul."

Then she added, "In our little town I had to be very careful not to say too much about anything religious. It was one of those places where there were deep tensions between majority Catholics and minority Protestants. I soon learned that this Lutheran coach better not say anything about religion. But nobody could fuss if I talked about the wonderful things that come from quiet—especially they wouldn't complain if we won."

═════

How could a girl so young (barely twenty) reach a level of spiritual maturity so deep, so wide, so fast?

I think I know one answer. All her life, Martha had been influenced by her mother's practice of the spiritual disciplines: reading her Bible, attending her church, ministering to needy neighbors and friends, sharing her love, but above all praying—talking to the Lord and listening.

For Martha, all this began early. How many times did I hear her say, "Every day before Herloff and I left for school, my mother would put her arms around us. Then she would say a prayer asking the Lord to bless us, to watch over the other children, to help our teachers, to give us all quick minds and loving hearts."

═════

Drop a stone into the water, and where will the ripples end? Say a prayer with your daughter, and how far does the spiritual influence flow? To a basketball team? To *those* girls' sons and daughters?

God alone knows the impact of one woman listening in the quiet, one woman teaching others of God's power and wisdom coming from the quiet.

"Shhh!"

MARRIAGE

If all the silent husbands of the world
were laid end to end, it would be a good
thing. Ditto for those occasional wives
who barricade themselves behind what
they should be sharing.
Charlie and Martha Shedd

———

Talk, Talk, Talk

If someone were to ask you, "What are the three most
important words in any marriage?" you might give one of
these answers:

"I love you."

"You are beautiful."

"Please forgive me."

All are excellent choices. But from our workshops, out of
letters we receive, in counseling sessions too, we've concluded
that the three most important words are:

"Talk! Talk! Talk!"

Why? Because without talk, talk, talk, "I love you" won't
get through. Neither will that all-important "You are beautiful" or the magic eraser, "Please forgive me."

Any way we come to it, heaven on earth is a relationship
in which two can say, "I want to know you, and I want you
to know me—no reservations." Any couple willing to make
that statement, and live by it, has arrived at the wellspring of
true love.

These were the opening words of Martha's presentation at
our Fun in Marriage workshops.

From there we would present together some of the techniques and precepts which had blessed us. The first two we called our "absolutes."

1. Absolute grace.   If I show you who I am and you don't like it, what do I have left? Nothing. Absolute grace is the divine attribute which says, "You can tell me anything. The times you were ashamed of yourself and the times you were proud, your dreams, your hopes, and even your wildest fantasies—I welcome them all.

"The more you tell me, the more I will love you, because I'll know you better. That is how God loves me, and that is how I love you.

"I pledge you the gift of absolute grace."

2. Absolute fidelity.   Physical faithfulness is a must. Without that, there can be no soul-security in any duo. But the same is true of things shared verbally.

"Therefore, I promise you also absolute secrecy about all you tell me, absolute loyalty when I talk about you in public. Whether you are with me or absent, I will be faithful."

Fidelity in every way is an absolute must.

========

To strengthen our "Talk! Talk! Talk!" commitment even further we also made two pledges.

Pledge One: Time for each other.   Those acquainted with our books know of our "weekly date" compact: an evening, lunch, or breakfast away from the family, apart from all others. This was our "date" alone to put elbows on the table and read each other's souls.

One couple we knew has what they call their Thursday afternoon matinee. He operates his own business, and Thursday, he says, "is for the most important business of my life."

A young wife writes, "For us it seems almost impossible to set aside time each week. So here's what we do: we have a weekend away together every month. Sure it takes planning, but you can't believe how much better things have gone between us since we started doing it. All month we look forward to it. This is when we really learn to know each other."

Any way it's done, it is one fine pledge: "We *will* make time for our togetherness. No matter what it requires, we *will* control our schedule. Our schedule will *not* control us."

Are we the only couple who almost always fussed a time or two when we had houseguests? Why these spats? We decided the reason was the interruption to our "one-ing." Amazing how much better it went after we adopted this little practice we came to love. Every time we had houseguests, we would go out to breakfast alone. On the kitchen table Martha would leave a pan of her pecan rolls. Beside them was a note: "Coffee ready. Have some of my rolls. Whenever we have houseguests, Charlie and I go out for breakfast alone. Thanks for coming."

Pledge Two: We will listen, listen, listen. We will listen with our ears and with our hearts. We will listen for the spoken and the unspoken.

Eight times Jesus said, "He that hath ears to hear, let him hear." (Phillips translation: "Pay attention to what you hear.") Why did He say it so often? Is it because we need it often? For some of us the answer is, "Yes, very often." Especially at home, some of us tend to forget our conversational manners.

It's a weighty pledge and hard to live by: "Listen. Listen. Listen."

=====

For us, the number one road to quality talking and quality listening was another commitment. This was our practice of regular Bible study and daily prayer with each other. But we also learned quickly that the little everyday sharings could make a mighty difference too.

One of these small blessings was
our covenant of compliments.

Every day an accolade—at least one "I like you because . . ." or "Have I told you how much I appreciate you?"

Blessed is the couple who remembers: Praise is like manna. It lasts only one day.

But the daily praise was only part of this covenant. Every week we paid each other a new compliment, something we'd never said before. Multiply fifty-two by the years you've been married. Does your mate know that many things you like?

Promise: If you will begin today (one compliment daily, one new compliment weekly) your marriage will take on a wonderful new glow. No small part of life's well-being comes from feeling that we're doing well. And nothing brings the heart more gladness than to know we're doing well with the person we love best. The Bible tells it like it is, "Love rejoices not at wrong but rejoices in the right" (1 Cor. 13).

Our second small blessing seems like an ordinary question, but with practice this can be a major toner too:

"What was your happiest moment today?"

With us it worked its magic best toward evening—mealtime, sitting time, bedtime. There are so many positives here:

Immediately we must begin reviewing the day. From all this day's good moments (surprising number), we select the very best. Here it is—my gift of a favorite memory for my favorite person this day.

Two absolutes. Two pledges. Two small blessings.

═════

The sad song of too many marriages is, "Where have all the flowers gone?" But it doesn't have to be this way. Those who learn to share all things both big and little will one day arrive where the blessed are.

Hear them saying it, feel them feeling it:

"Lucky, lucky us. However did it happen that the two most interesting people on earth should come together in our marriage?"

When she speaks, her words are wise,
and kindness is the rule for everything
she says.

Proverbs 31:26, LB

Critique, with the Fun Touch

Does the Lord equip some of his favorites with special radar for things most of us miss? Or is it that these folks are more tuned in to His blessings than others? "More tuned in" must be nearer to the truth than "favorites."

As I watched Martha living her "tuned to the Inner Presence" life, this came clear. She was sensitive to beautiful thoughts and ideas. Where others only walked, she'd feel a certain pull. Then, scratching around a bit, she might come up with buried treasure. Or if it was only a piece of trivia, no matter. With it she would spend a few minutes loitering around in her imagination.

This tendency was particularly interesting as I shared my sermons and writings with her.

You can believe she thought I was a cut above average. Yet she never got so carried away that she couldn't control her adoration. "I will try" she would say, "to listen as though I might be someone who never heard of you."

Try, she did, and she succeeded. Any seminary would have been fortunate to have her. In their chair of homiletics (the art of preaching) she'd have done wonders. One of America's leading publishers many times told her, "If anything should happen to Charlie, you come see us. We will immediately install you as one of our senior editors." Whenever he said that, she would smile her "See, you better be good to me" smile. And I would flash back, "Never you worry, I will."

Every week a sermon; regularly the newspaper columns, speeches, books, magazine articles. All of them I'd bring to the kiln of her critique.

Martha was an avid reader. Prayer and the mystics, fiction and nonfiction, poetry and prose, history, biography, detective stories, mystery tales, the humorous and the serious—all were her terrain. And always she read with her radar turned on, especially turned on for things to share with me. She was an absolute genius too at picking up wisdom sayings that would apply to my preaching. And she was especially fond of items with humorous shading, sly or not so sly.

Example: When I was spending too much time on the unimportant; if I was fussing over some peccadillo; she might quote me this from a mystic of the Middle Ages:

"I think right here, Charlie, you may be burning down the cathedral to fry an egg."

———

Not all of Martha's rememberables came from her reading. Sometimes it seemed to me God whispered in her ear exactly the right advice at exactly the right time. An example: On occasions when I was into one of the ministerial days of over-say (writers also have these days), she would let me soar for a time. Then when enough was enough she would say, "That is beautiful, Charlie. Absolutely beautiful. But what do you want me to do about it?"

This was so like Martha. Decorations she enjoyed, but never over-decorating. Since all God's children got troubles these days she wanted her preacher to keep it practical, keep it helpful. Toward which end she often added this favorite saying, "Why put ruffles on the stars?"

=====

If I could retain only one favorite of all my Martha adages, this would be it—her rendition of some sage advice via one small-town depot.

George was the Union Pacific Railroad agent at Lexington, Nebraska. Only a few of the natives could remember when he hadn't been there. Most of them had been blessed by his presence, and I had too.

I never should have gone to Lexington when I did. A church of seven hundred needed someone much wiser than me. Yet here I was, trying hard, making mistakes, and running to George for help.

On a particular day I had come to the depot with another parish problem. A certain prominent businessman had been reelected to the church board. No one was happy about it, including me. This man was big trouble for us all—cantankerous, down on everything. So why was he back in office? Because he had been serving on and off for years; he controlled the bank which held our building loan; and he was a significant giver.

I had been warned about him, but, being young and inexperienced, my attitude was, "Never fear, Charlie is here." I would win him over. Give me a few months. I'd be nice to him, spend time with him, love him. Gradually I would remake him. He and I would become best friends.

No sale. The man did not want friends. I suppose at one time down the dim corridors of his past he must have hoped someone would love him. But not now, and not this preacher. Try as I might, it was the same song, next verse: "Go away.

Leave me alone. I happen to like being everybody's nuisance. Yours too."

So I had come to counsel with George. He was busy when I arrived, but no matter. I always enjoyed watching his hands at the telegraph keys. How many words per minute could he do? Many, many.

When he had finished his message, he invited me behind the No Admittance gate. "Have a seat. Want some coffee? You look down. Something bothering you?"

Something was indeed bothering me, and I told him. I was about to give up on Mr. X. "Do you have any suggestions for me, George? Has he ever been different? Ever been nice? What can I do?"

To my questions came the same monotonous answers: "No!" "No!" "No!" and "Nothing!" And then that day I was to hear one of the most significant speeches I ever heard— short, clear, message unmistakable. I often wondered if George hadn't prepared this speech. Knowing him and his super Sunday school lessons, he might have. Did he also rehearse it, knowing I'd be in for it some day? That was possible too.

"Charlie," he began, "I've been watching you. You've given it your best, and that's not good enough. The man is miserable, and the only satisfaction he gets is making the rest of us miserable. He's never liked any of our preachers, and he'll never like you. But not everyone liked Jesus, remember? He lost one out of twelve. Better face it, son. Comparing you with Jesus, maybe you'll do well to *hold* one out of twelve."

You can believe I went straight home from the depot that day. Monumental moments like this are for sharing.

Martha and I laughed and laughed. Right then George's classic became one of our all-time favorites. And reworked by Martha it became something else. This was exactly what she'd been needing for her young preacher husband. He may have been called to the ministry, all right, but of this she was sure—the Lord had not called him to remake the world.

"Charlie," she said, "that is plain vanilla wonderful. Great new saying straight from the Source:

"Never try to out-Jesus Jesus."

It is the little rift within the lute that by
and by will make the music mute.

Tennyson

Seven Official Rules for a Good, Clean Fight

Dear Charlie:
I hate you.
Love,
martha

She may have been the first to say it. That I do not know.
What I do know is that it blew my hair back. It had never
occurred to me that this loving woman I'd married could also
hate me.

It was a handwritten note, sealed in an envelope, on top
of my sandwich. Martha made super sandwiches. Usually we
ate our evening meal together, but tonight she was at her
young mothers' prayer group. This was a covered-dish dinner,
a beautiful array of young, young mothers eager to learn from
their pastor's wife. They knew she knew some things they
needed to know about prayer.

As I opened the envelope, I fully expected one of her
loving notes, full of affection, full of promise. But what a
shocker. She hated me!

I knew what incited the note, and looking back I knew too that I had it coming. (I still think it may have been a little bit her fault.) But "hate"? Really?

Yes, really!

So what's the matter with that? Nothing at all if it moves toward a deeper love. Nothing at all if it clears the inner chambers of latent troublemakers.

"Rules for a Good, Clean Fight" we called our covenants for disagreement. Together we hammered them out. Right then we accepted this fact: wherever two red-blooded people are building a home, there will be occasional spats and, now and then, some fiery encounter.

When we accepted this fact, then we could begin shaping some specific agreements for disagreement.

So here now are the Charlie and Martha "Seven Official Rules for a Good, Clean Fight." We signed them in our souls as affirmations. I give them to you just as we enjoyed them (well, not always, but mostly) for forty-eight years.

1. Before We Begin, We Must Both Agree That the Time is Right.

There is this eager little beaver in nearly every one of us: "Something is needling me. Let's get right on with it." But some days it takes all our strength just to go on breathing. So the wise woman learns to purr with the kittens at times when she would prefer to scratch with the cats. And the smart man learns how to back off when he would like to attack.

Some things better wait. Some things should not wait. Some things might wait too long. Whatever we do, we both better make certain we know the bailiff's two questions, "Is the defendant ready?" and "Is the plaintiff prepared?"

2. We Will Remember That Our Only Battle Aim is a Deeper Understanding of Each Other.

There are several important gun labels for conversational warfare between husbands and wives who really do care.

"Patience" is one for sure. Without it we could tear up more in an hour than it might take weeks to repair.

"Mercy," "grace," and "telling the truth in love" should be in our hearts as we shout, "Ready, aim, fire!"

Say it one more time. Our main aim is to improve this marriage by deeper understanding!

3. We Will Check Our Weapons Often to be Sure They're Not Deadly.

This rule follows naturally on the heels of the first two. "The battle unto death" may be all right in its place, but its place is not in the home. Here we are shooting down troubles, not firing for funerals!

So we must be especially careful of the words we hurl when the smoke gets in our eyes.

Major warning here: Cruelty is bad in any form, and one of the worst is to throw up to others those things they can never change.

Another weapon to lay aside permanently is overused phrases which have become tiresome: "You are *never* home on time!" "You *always* put the children first!" These and their ilk only ignite fuses and lead to trouble. We will strive to delete "never" and "always" from our battle vocabulary.

Now comes a paradox! There are times when no answer is the best answer. But at other times it may be worse to say nothing than to say something. Utter absence of any utterance from the person we love most can be strictly no good. If we're dying for our mate to break the silence, that silence may be one of the loudest noises ever heard.

The swords we swing on this "battle of the bridge" must be cut of stuff that bends and gives. Our cannonballs should be more like snowballs than great balls of fire.

4. *We Will Lower Our Voices Instead of Raising Them.*

This rule of our seven was built into our courtship before we married. It came, like so many good things of our love, from out of Martha's quiet. In my stormy background we "hollered" when our ire was up. And always the volume went higher with increasing ire.

When Martha and I began our dating, I sensed what Shakespeare meant when he said, "Her voice was ever soft, gentle, and low, an excellent thing in woman"!

But as it does with all sweethearts, the first hour of anger arrived, and I began my customary shouting. She stopped me in my vocal tracks and explained her better way. "Why don't we agree," she said from her inner stillness, "that from now on when we fuss, we'll lower our voices one octave rather than raising them two?" Rule 4 for us rates the title "Cardinal Rule."

5. *We Will Never Quarrel in Public or Reveal Private Matters.*

Conversation heard often from certain types:

"On the first Tuesday it rained, so we stayed in the cabin and played cards!"

"No! No! No! Don't you remember, darling, on Tuesday we drove over the mountain. Wednesday was the day it rained!"

"It was Tuesday; it had to be Tuesday because . . ."

To this there is only one proper piece of advice: "Why don't you two do your dirty laundry at home?"

Rule: All rubbing and scrubbing of laundry should be done in its place, and its place is in private!

There is one subpoint to this rule. We also agree that we will never fire at each other publicly when we are not together. (Another rule to underscore with heavy red pencil.)

6. We Will Discuss an Armistice Whenever Either of Us Calls "Halt."

Notice the wording, "We will *discuss* an armistice!" Some people are quitters by nature. They run up the white flag too soon! Sometimes silence is not golden; it may be a pale shade of yellow.

How can we end it if we want to quit and our adversary wants to continue? Here is one move for cease-fire that seldom fails. It goes like this, "I'm beginning to see what you mean! But I'll need some time to think this over. Please, let's make up now so I can consider awhile how you could be right!"

7. When We Have Come to Terms, We Will Put it Away Until We Both Agree it Needs More Discussing.

A healthy union requires that we never forget some things and never remember others. Wedlock must have its lockboxes. In some of these we must put certain items and throw the key away. Others we keep for later opening.

Now back to Martha's note. Nice sandwich. Message not so nice, but oh so necessary. Love and hate *can* rendezvous in the same mind. And if left there unnoticed, unattended, unseparated, one day we know the truth of that old mountain saying: "If we don't carry out the garbage, one day our house becomes a dump."

Or, say it one more time with the literary touch, "It is the little rift within the lute that by and by may make the music mute."

Errors, like straws, upon the
   surface flow;
He who would search for pearls
   must dive below.
                              Dryden

Loving the Unlovable

We had stopped at an all-night restaurant. It was two in the morning and not our best hour. So why were we here? We were on our way home from a speaking engagement in Tulsa.

The waitress that night was an attractive young woman. She actually looked out of place here. And this obviously was not her best time either. No greeting. None whatsoever. She was brusque, bordering on rude. She took our order and served us grudgingly. She had left off an item or two, but we let it go, too tired to hassle.

During the early years of our marriage, Martha was quite reserved in public. She would smile, would speak when spoken to, but almost never initiated a conversation. On rare occasions, though, she would surprise me with a departure from the usual. So now, as the waitress took our dishes and brought dessert—no one else in the restaurant—Martha reached out, touched the girl's hand, and said, "You're having a hard night, aren't you? Anything we can do for you?"

The young woman stopped and stood still as a statue. She looked at both of us. I think she was seeing us for the first time.

Then she began sobbing, and here came a flood of tears. From way down in her breaking heart, she cried her story.

That very day, she said, she had been served papers from her husband's lawyer. He wanted a divorce. No, she hadn't expected this action. She knew that in recent months, maybe a year, things hadn't been what they used to be. Yet she'd been giving her best, and she honestly thought their marriage might be improving a little. Now he had opted for the other woman, and the marriage was all over. What could she do?

Four little children, and however would she be able to support them alone? Her mother worked; her grandmother wasn't well. How could she afford a baby-sitter? This waitress job, she said, was an extra. She was a secretary during the day and a good one. But how long could she go on being good at anything with all she had to do?

Her rent was due, and she must keep working. How could she carry on with so little rest? How? How? Why? Why? What if? And on and on.

Of course we tried to help her, as you would. Then because we asked her, she gave us her name, address, phone number. For a long time we stayed in touch. Finally she married again. Fine man, she said he was. Wouldn't you think so? Noble soul, taking on one wife, four children. Lord give them a happy ending.

As we left the restaurant that night, now past three, we were both quiet. Then selecting from her thoughts, Martha said, "If only we could remember when people aren't nice to us, it's because someone hasn't been nice to them. I'm glad we didn't give her a hard time back."

So was I. It would have spoiled one of the memorable agreements of our marriage. At first we didn't write it, except on our hearts. Then, because we described it often in our workshops, requests came for written copies. We called it

Our Pledge for Loving the Unlovable

> Whenever you are not at your best,
>> if you will let me,
>>> I will put my arms around you
>>> and hold you close.
> Then while I am holding you, I promise
>> I will try to keep my cool when you are angry.
>> I will try to be soft when you are hard.
>> I will try to act rather than react.
> If you will listen, I will promise you:
>> even when you are down on life
>> down on me, down on yourself
>>> I will be up on the basic you.
> Here, now and forever
> I will do my best to love the unlovable.

======

I like to begin premarital consultations by asking the prospective bride and groom, "What do you like best about each other?" Easy. Almost immediately, here come the accolades: "I just love everything about him." "I can't think of one single thing I don't like about her."

To which there can only be one answer. "You come back in six months, and we'll discuss it again." Some of them do come, and always—no exception—there is adequate data now for further consideration.

They say that love is blind, and it is, which may be a very good thing. Up to a point it may be a good thing. Then again, that blindness can't go on forever. Some day, sometime in our love, we must face this one stiff fact: we are united to an imperfect human being, imperfect at least for perfect union with us.

When we married, Martha and I were operating under the delusion that ours was the perfect union. But on the first morning of our honeymoon that delusion came to a great lurch. *Our sleeping timers were irrevocably different.*

The scenario went like this:

ME: Early morning riser. Early. Early.
SHE: Late morning sleeper. The later the better.
ME: Early to bed. Come, put it away.
SHE: The exact opposite.

I truly think the Lord had equipped Martha with some delicate "after-supper antenna." Dishes were done. Darkness descended. Here came the bulletins of her night: Knit an afghan. Braid a rug. Read a book. Call a friend. Go for a walk.

For forty-eight years that's how it went. And the conversations for forty-eight years went something like this: "Oh, Charlie, do you *have* to get up so early?"

"Do *you* have to put the stars away?"

"But you don't even believe in God, Martha, till 8:30 in the morning and two cups of coffee."

Certainly we tried to make adjustments. We experimented. We even took turns being miserable in our attempts to live by each other's clocks. Always the same result: I would wish she'd stayed asleep. She would pry me out of my chair, walk me to the bedroom, tuck me in.

For forty-eight years it was never any different. As far as the east is from the west, so far our timers were set apart.

There were other differences too, some mendable, some not. You wouldn't want me to share all the strife and friction in our love. Ours was ours, and yours is yours. Private.

Did I say there was nothing we could do about the timers? That's not quite true. Martha had an appropriate little speech she would make on occasion. It was a speech just for the two of us, varied as needed, and I loved it. "You know," she'd begin, "this is something I learned in home economics. When you braid a rug or knit a sweater, there will be flaws in it. When you finish a piece of furniture or make something for your home, same thing. There will be flaws in that too.

"But here is an amazing principle: If you don't let the flaws upset you too much, if you keep what you've made long enough, if you give it a chance, a wonderful thing happens. One day the flaws will blend right in. They make it unique. They actually help to make it beautiful. Then you will love it."

It was a good speech, accompanied by a very nice ritual. When she was through, we would nod our heads and smile. After that we would talk a bit about how that applied to everything, including us.

Then these two imperfect creatures of the perfect Lord would hold each other. So close we would hold each other, and be ever so grateful, grateful that we had learned so much about loving the unlovable, in things, in life, and in each other.

When the one man loves the one woman
And the one woman loves the one man,
The very angels leave heaven
And come and sit in that house
And sing for joy.

Anonymous

========

Prevenient Grace

Seven years is a long time for knowing. And shouldn't seven years of courtship be enough? Seven years to get acquainted, to share, to talk, to learn, to know some more, to love and fuss and love again. Shouldn't that be long enough to eliminate potential problems?

Sounds reasonable, but it wasn't long enough for us!

"Jealousy" is an ugly word with an ugly sound, but it's even uglier in reality. In reality jealousy can do marriage in, and that is what it might have done to us, except for Martha.

I am a hugger, a public hugger. "Hail, hail, the gang's all here! Let us love one another with whole heart fervently."

Martha was a hugger too, but with this difference. She was a hugger of one—me! Dignified, quiet, shy—the slow approach.

Then why hadn't we sensed the dormant problem lurking here? Why is it that certain sinister threats come on padded feet?

I was a young pastor and in over my head, serving a church too large for one so young. But I was loving the flock, and the flock was loving me. A good combination, unless the young pastor isn't very good yet at reading inner feelings.

In every church there are women—single women, unhappily married women, women of every size, every shape. And some of them think their new minister is the finest thing out. What is he like personally, they wonder—meaning close up? So they come for counseling appointments, program appointments, officer appointments, committee appointments. They come for help with their Church School lessons. They come too seeking help with their marriage. If they're not married they come for help with that. It's busy work for the new pastor, and interesting.

Because you're getting nervous, as I am, I should tell you now. I was never unfaithful to Martha in the traditional sense of unfaithful as a husband. Unfaithful, yes, in thought sometimes, unfaithful in understanding, unfaithful in caring enough.

So it was largely my fault that she was jealous. She knew the women were big fans of her husband. She also knew why some of them felt as they felt. She knew too that I was basking in all these accolades, all this attention. Basking too much. And I, not caring enough that she cared so much, handled the whole thing badly. "Jealous wives—these we have always with us. Sorry fellows, that's how they are. So, forget it. Hug on!"

This attitude unchecked could plainly lead to disaster. For everyone, including the Lord who had brought us together, it could lead to disaster.

All this, as you surmise, was strictly no good. No good for many reasons, not least of which was a slow erosion in our love. I didn't like it, and she didn't. She really was my favorite, and I really was hers. What could we do?

She decided there was one thing she could do. She could take it to the Lord in prayer. No one knew there were storm clouds gathering at the manse, but she knew. So she prayed: "Dear Lord, before anything happens to scar our memories, or scar the church, enfold this whole thing in Your love. Purify the air between us, purge our minds of dangerous attitudes; heal, correct, save us."

Then, in true Martha spirit, I'm sure she added, "Lord, love through me. You show me what to do, and I will do it."

That was so much like Martha. Sometimes she prayed at length. Sometimes she made quick prayers. But always her prayers were straight to the point, and so many times that's how the answers came back. Straight. To the point.

Living with this and watching it happen, I often wondered, Had the Lord told His secretary, "If it's a call from Martha, I'll take it"?

That very evening (she said it was the same day she'd heard the Lord's answer) she met me at the door wearing a pretty apron, my favorite dress, a loving smile. "Today, Charlie," she announced, "I have reached a big decision, and I will tell you all about it. Only first I will feed you. Come to dinner." (Great idea. Any time you're about to lay something major on him, feed him. Prelude the whole thing with one of his favorite dinners.)

So, once we'd fared well together, she began, "Charlie, about that big decision. You know I don't like what's been happening between us, and you know why. I've been jealous, that's why, and it's strange, because I do feel I can trust you. Yet I've been so afraid—afraid that you with all your love and affection might someday get involved where you shouldn't in a way you shouldn't. And what would I do then?

"What could I do now? I could pray. So I prayed, and the Lord showed me what to do. Now I will do it. I am telling you that no matter what you do, I will never stop loving you. Never, not ever. I hope you don't ever have an affair, Charlie. I think it would kill something inside me. But I would forgive you, and I wouldn't quit loving you. I know what I'm saying, Charlie, and I mean it. This is the truth. Even while you're having that affair, I'll be right there in the wings loving you, forgiving you. That is how much I love you!"

How could a man ever be unfaithful to a love like that? For one man I know the answer is, "He couldn't!"

━━━━

Our catechism says, "Grace is the free, unmerited love and favor of God." Beautiful affirmation, theology at its finest, except possibly for one addendum. "Prevenient grace" is the addendum, meaning different things to different scholars. But could it ever have any more perfect meaning than this?

Grace in all its fullness
   flowing through the heart of a woman
      so in tune with the divine
that she too can love
   without limits
      ahead of time.

Here is my description of a truly happy
land where Jehovah is God: Sons vigorous
and tall as growing plants. Daughters of
graceful beauty.

Psalm 144:12, LB

"There Hain't No Way"

Among life's nonnegotiables is the fact that we're all getting older every twenty-four hours. That may be one reason
Grandma Shepherd was so much fun. She made us feel we
could hardly wait to get as old as she was. Interesting. Entertaining. So alive.

She had come to our church in Oklahoma to be near her
daughter. Practical as she was, she'd agreed with her family.
At this stage of her life she should live closer to some relative.
So here she was, straight out of the Missouri hills, full of
stories, everybody's pet.

Among our favorites was her tale of the young preacher's
sermon on parenting. It happened, she said, in the tiny church
where she grew up.

"We couldn't afford a full-time preacher, but whenever
we could we'd have what we called a supply. Sometimes they
didn't supply much, but one year we were lucky. A young
student came from the seminary, and he was a dandy. Only
sometimes he got in over his head. But we didn't mind. He
wasn't married, so all of us girls thought he was especially
promising.

"On this particular Sunday he announced, 'Today, folks,
I'm going to preach on how to raise your children.' This was

a small church, remember, right informal, and all kinds of characters among us.

"Well, when the preacher announced he would talk about raising children, an old mountain grandma from back in the sanctuary said aloud, 'There hain't no way, Reverend. There just hain't no way.'"

Grandma Shepherd never told us what happened next. But don't you suppose every parent in that little mountain church felt like saying a loud amen?

Martha and I would have joined in. Four sons and one daughter do not an expert make. We never thought of ourselves as experts, but we gave it all we had.

═══════

"What would you do if you could raise your children again?" "Looking back, what mistakes do you think you made, and how would you correct them this time?" Often here came the "what if" questions. They came so regularly we did some serious reconnoitering and prepared a list.

Here now is a brief look at the answers. In all honesty, they really aren't answers. They are instead a review of things we'd do again if we were parents once more. May you find them helpful, but if you don't, remember the old mountain grandma.

1. The First Thing We'd Do Again Is to Set Aside Time for Togetherness.   Around the dinner table every night we would share "interesting things." We would open our hearts to each other. Laughing, crying, arguing, complaining, we would "coalesce," as Martha liked to call it. We would also repeat this time-sharing event: monthly, each child would have one night out alone with Dad.

2. We Would Let Our Children Vote on Matters Affecting the Whole Family.   Democracy is not taught by saluting the flag or singing "The Star-Spangled Banner." By making motions, discussing, and voting, several important things are learned: self-respect ("my opinion does count"), respect for the rights of others ("their opinion counts too"), appreciation of the way our country runs, appreciation for a mother and father who recognize both their children's rights and their children's intelligence.

3. We Would Set Some Specific Boundaries for Behavior.
"Here are the fences, children. Beyond these we do not go." Rules and regulations, penalties and rewards—all these we'll discuss and clarify. Group control, yes, but the goal is self-control. Discipline, yes, but here too the aim is self-discipline. Good behavior expected. Bad behavior punished.

4. We Would Have a Challenging, Well-Worked-Out, Fun System for Allowances.   One of our favorite baby-sitters, sometime cook, sometime maid was fond of saying, "You don't get nothin' for nothin' but nothin'." That, children, is true around here.

5. We Would Emphasize Moral Education, Drug Education, Sex Education, Alcohol Education, and How to Say No, Loudly, Clearly, Often.   The laws of the land, the laws of God, and "Thus saith the Lord" (church, Sunday school, religious training—all nonoptional). In the face of cults, devil worship, abnormal behavior, and the bizarre, how do today's parents make it? Carefully, prayerfully, constantly alert—that's how.

6. We Would Worship at Home as a Family.   If we were parents again, and we could choose only one thing to repeat, this would be it—our "Fun Family Devotions." Every evening at dinner "interesting things" would be followed by a Bible reading or devotional selection. These would be chosen by the evening leader. Then prayer time—sentence prayers, silent prayer, prayer by the leader, and the Lord's Prayer together. Always the same goals: fun, interesting, daily, all intended to help us remember one important truth—the real altar of God is this altar in our home and in our hearts.

———

Why all this effort to be effective in our parenting? Why even think about what we'd do if we were doing it again?

Isn't *this* the real reason, the reason of the wisdom writer? "Your children are not your children. They come through you but not from you." (Kahlil Gibran)

So right, isn't he?
For us as the Lord's believers,
parenting *is* the all-important business
of preparing *His* children
to be what *He* intended
for *Him.*

PASTOR'S WIFE

The church will win the world for Christ
when—and only when—she works
through living spirits steeped in prayer.
Evelyn Underhill

————————

The Praying Church and a
Pastor's Praying Wife

Memorial Drive Presbyterian Church in Houston, Texas, is a powerhouse of spiritual energy: six thousand members worshiping, praying, serving, giving. "Giving" as in matching dollars—a dollar to missions for every dollar spent on local needs. Programs, salaries, supplies, utilities, miscellaneous—all matched dollar for dollar.

Martha and I had the fun of launching "MDPC," as Memorial Drive Presbyterian is affectionately known. Thirty-five years ago we moved from Oklahoma to "the throbbing city on the Bayou." No way it made sense for us to leave a church of fifteen hundred for someone else's dream, minus guarantees. But we went, and it was exciting.

Every week hundreds of new residents were pouring into Houston, moving into new homes springing up everywhere—on the prairie, among the trees with their Spanish moss—row on row of new homes. Street names like Sleepy Oaks, Butterfly Lane, Mossy Cup, Misty Meadow, Piping Rock. Suddenly here were all these people, and here we were on a strategic corner with a sign that read

Come, let us worship together
at Spring Branch Junior High.

We met at the school because our only building was an old house in a pasture. Dubbed "Charlie's shed" by some wag in our congregation, it had once been a worthy farmhouse. But now, rickety, worn, hard to heat, barely holding together, "shed" was a fitting label. It was a collection of old boards among all those posh new houses, houses selling fast, filling up fast.

Fast too were the new cars hurrying by us twice daily. Every morning, banners flying, speeding to their fine offices, fine jobs, fine futures. Then in the evening here they came again, banners dragging a bit now, most of them weary. Wistful, wondering.

What are they wondering?

"Isn't there something better than this, Jane? Sure, we're making a living, but what are we making of our lives?"

"The children, John. Are we doing too much *for* them but not enough *with* them?"

"Suppose we ought to try church again? Remember our church in Connecticut? The friends we made there, the music, the things we learned? Such a caring church. Remember?"

"Didn't I see something about a church at the junior high? Think we should give it a look?"

So they gave our church a look, and the serious gave it another look.

At its heart were two dynamic programs, real dynamos of spiritual power. First, the matching of dollars spent at home with dollars to missions. Second, the commitment to prayer. Every member in the church was prayed for every day by some other member.

———

A church where everyone would be prayed for daily had been a new idea to me. But that's what they wanted, so naturally they turned to their leader. And I'm ashamed to admit that right then an old couplet crossed my mind:

When diving and finding no pearls in the sea;
Blame not the ocean, the fault is in thee.

What can a man do when he's on the spot and he doesn't know what he should know? Sure, I could tell them the whole idea of a praying church was altogether new to me. But should I also confess how little I knew personally about prayer?

That's what I decided to do. I confessed, and I was surprised. They didn't panic. Was this because they didn't understand what they were asking? Or had they already decided they had called a minor prophet to be their pastor? What can you expect of a minor prophet?

What I told them was that I did know one person who knew a lot about prayer. That's where I would go for help.

I did not tell them who she was. She wouldn't have liked that. But I was right.

She *did* have some answers.

Where two or three are gathered together
in my name, there am I in the midst of
them.

Matthew 18:20, KJV

The Chapel in Our Love

This is a confession I would rather not make, but it has
to be made. It has to be made here for two reasons: First,
without it I couldn't explain the cataclysmic alterations necessary in the new pastor of that new church in Houston. The
second reason I must own up to my barren soul is that if I do,
you will better understand Martha. Almost more than any
other episode in our relationship, what happens now reflects
the gentle Martha spirit to perfection.

So, on to the awful truth: I was a minister for some years
before I came to know the Lord personally. That isn't to say
I was unsuccessful as a pastor. I didn't disgrace the church.
Neither my denomination nor the local congregations I served
were ever embarrassed by Charlie. On the contrary, I was a
roaring success in many ways.

When I finished seminary, I set my sights for the top. Mine
would be rapid advancement, recognition, and a big church.
So by earthly standards I was on my way. Smooth. Clever.
Professional. See the man go.

But where was he going, and why?

During all these years I loved my wife. More than anything I loved her. I liked so many things about her, and one
of the things I liked best was what she did in the morning.

When she'd had her coffee and her world was no longer a gray mass, always she made the same little pilgrimage. Gathering her books, her Bible, paper, pen, and pencil, she'd head for her own special corner. I named that corner "Martha's Sanctuary," and that's what it was for her. There she was alone in her own native world. Not quite accurate, that last line. She wasn't alone, because the Lord was there and she was tuning in to Him—studying His Book, asking Him to teach her, reading her devotional literature. Thinking, praying, drawing on energies I never even knew were there.

This I liked for many reasons, and one is that it gave me a sense of security, a solid feeling. Perhaps there was even a touch of that "My uncle was a preacher" line. Every pastor hears it, said usually with a touch of the hopeful, as in, "Don't worry about me, Reverend. My uncle was a preacher."

Not being into prayer myself, I did have shades of that feeling as I watched her in her sanctuary. When I was away from home and I pictured her there, the very thought seemed to support me. When now and then she told me about the goings-on between herself and the Lord, I liked that too. It made me feel that if I ever did want to get serious about serious things, I'd know where to go for starters.

Now the time had arrived. I'd been brought to that moment when I was empty of ideas, empty of cleverness, empty of soul. No young preacher's snow job would do it now. They wanted to know, "How do we start a praying church?" Did Martha have any answers?

═══════

She had always been interested in prayer. From childhood on, Martha had been trained to pray. "Sounds wonderful," she said. "A church where every member is prayed for every day.

Absolutely marvelous. Let's begin. All we need is the idea. If we take step one, the Lord will show us step two."

And He did.

But that first step wasn't what I thought it would be. I will never forget that day. I was sitting there on the floor in front of her.

"Martha," I began, "they want a praying church. Will you help me? I feel so empty. I don't know anything about prayer."

The angels must have been bending low to hear her answer. What would she say? "I've known all along you're a bit of a con man, Charlie. But if you really mean business, I'll share my knowledge with you."

Any one of a dozen lectures she might have given me, and I'd have deserved them all. But what she did say wasn't anything like that. It was one of the most beautiful invitations I've ever heard.

Almost in a whisper she said, "Charlie, nobody knows much about prayer, including me. Prayer is like a journey. Every path you take leads to another gate, another door. Let's explore together. This could be the most wonderful day of our lives. The day we became prayer partners. A wonderful, wonderful day."

═══

Most couples who have tried praying together will bump into one cold, hard fact: developing a turned-on, tuned-in prayer life for husband and wife is much easier said than done.

When we first began, there were many awkward moments, but none more awkward than our initial attempts to pray with each other.

A couple beginning to pray with each other may wonder, "What if I tell the Lord what I'm really thinking, and my wife doesn't like it?" "If I surface my feelings aloud, will my husband understand?" "Should I share all my thoughts?" "All this makes me nervous."

To which comes the loud answering chorus: "Say it for us too. We felt that way. It was too scary, too sensitive, too embarrassing."

Can this be the reason why, in any survey we've ever taken, less than 5 percent of married couples actually pray together with meaning? That statistic includes Christian couples, church couples.

So there had to be a better way, and we found one.

Silent Prayer Together

1. We would sit hand in hand on our love seat and discuss our concerns.
2. We'd share the things we wanted to pray for.
3. Still holding hands, together in perfect quiet, we'd make our way to what we liked to call "the chapel in our love." Here we would pray silently, pray about the things we had shared together.
4. Then, when one of us felt it right, we'd conclude with the Lord's Prayer. Sometimes it might be the Twenty-third Psalm or another favorite before the amen.

How long did it take until praying aloud became natural? Not long for some themes. For others, never.

To the very end of Martha's life we prayed some days in silence. To every couple there come times, which the Scripture describes as "groanings of the spirit." When we were dealing with nebulous things, shadowy things—often we would pray them through silently. And somehow in the silence they seemed a bit more bearable through prayer.

So here's a prediction: Any couple not now praying together who will set aside time each day for silent prayer will experience improvement in every aspect of their relationship. And when the end comes for one of them, blessed are they who have been together often at the chapel of prayer in their love.

———

Question:

How do we start a praying church?

Answer from the pastor's wife:

The praying church starts at the chapel

in our hearts,

in our home,

in our love.

From people who pray we must become
people who bless.

Nietzsche

After-note on a
Praying Church

Memorial Drive Presbyterian in Houston is still a
bellwether church—bellwether as in leader, guide, forward
mover. Annual Budget 1990: $3 million; $1.5 million for local
needs, $1.5 million to missions.

Its current pastor, Dr. Tommy Tewell, is Mr. Enthusiasm.
A dynamic preacher, a leader par excellence, a lover—lover
of wife, lover of flock, lover of the Lord. It's a lucky, lucky
church to be led by such a leader. "Fortunate" is a better word.
"Divine guidance" describes it even better.

Divine guidance now and way back there at the beginning—that's the explanation. As I look back in review, this
truth comes clear to me: without Martha's love, without her
knowledge of prayer, Memorial Drive Church would never
have become what it became. I was the pastor out front,
looking far better than I really was. But I had a source. I was
drawing strength from a spiritual powerhouse.

Behind the scenes, Martha: Giving generously to missions,
helping lead that first little cluster to fifty-fifty giving. Praying, teaching others to pray (including her favorite pupil—
me), guiding prayer groups, organizing the membership for
intercessory prayer. Quiet, never much in the public eye, but
always there tending the dynamos, especially tending these

two dynamos: dollar-for-dollar giving, member-for-member praying.

Lucky, lucky church in their present pastor. Lucky, lucky too in their first mistress of the manse. Yes, "fortunate," "blessed" are the better words. But more than any other words, these from the Book tell it like it is. Always with the best of leaders it can be said, "Thou art come to the kingdom for such a time as this" (Esther 4:14, kjv).

Test everything.
Hold on to the good.
1 Thessalonians 5:21, NIV

———

Tests for Spiritual Growth

How can we be sure our prayer life is authentic? Is there any way we can know for certain what is real and what is not?

When Martha and I started praying together, we also began reading what others said about prayer. There is a vast collection of literature on prayer. Many writings too address spiritual life in general. There are also books, articles, pamphlets on living with the Lord daily, hourly. One well-known writer even presents his thoughts on minute-by-minute checks for divine contact.

Martha had already traveled down some of these roads. Her library of favorites was there for me. To these we added new titles that appealed to us. In libraries and bookstores we browsed and selected. Most of the time we were not reading together. We did give it a good try, but our timers simply would not synchronize.

So I got up early and had my own quiet time. I read, studied, prayed, meditated exactly as she had taught me. Today I still do it her way, with few variations. For me, Martha had it going exactly as it should be.

Still, both of us kept checking for authenticity. The many roads of prayer led many different ways. Some of them were exactly what we needed. But some led to twilight zones too far out for us.

Where could we find some absolute measurements, authentic gauges for being sure? We couldn't find them in the literature, so we decided to work out our own tests.

———

When I was in junior high, I candled eggs at the grocery across our street. For ten cents an hour I was employed to save the buyer from bad eggs. Or to put it positively, I was paid to make sure the buyers got what they paid for.

I sat on a stool. Before me was a small box with a hole on top. Inside was a light bulb. Each egg from the farmer's wife had to be carefully lifted and held over the hole to make certain it was good. Good eggs were clear, but dark spots meant this egg was about to spoil.

Galatians 5:22–23 is what Martha and I called "the great egg candler of the Bible." By these verses we could test our own progress in prayer—no mistaking. We could also judge the real in any writing, any movement, any group, any speaker. Individually by these tests we would know whether we were on solid ground. Even the church, its programs and leaders, its prayer efforts—all of it could be tested here. Then we discovered another thing. If we put all the aspects of our marriage up against the light here, we could candle our love too.

From this passage we worked out our nine tests, egg candlers straight from Galatians 5:22–23: "The fruit of the spirit is love, joy, peace, long-suffering, gentleness, goodness, faith, meekness, temperance" (KSV).

Important note: the word is "fruit," not "fruits." So what does that mean? It means we are not the producers. Love, joy, peace, and all these other fine qualities are by-products of life with the Lord.

Here then are the nine tests for spiritual growth Martha and I developed for ourselves. The extra words included with each test are selected from other translations of Galatians 5:22–23 or from our dictionaries.

1. The Fruit of the Spirit Is Love.

Is there an increasing concern for each other in our marriage?

More and more do we really care what our mate thinks and feels?

Are we growing in our "otherness"?

From other sources, more words for love:
charity, caring, concern, solicitude, devotion.

2. The Fruit of the Spirit Is Joy.

Are there increasing seasons of gladness in our relationship?

Are there more times when we sense the glow of real happiness, when we just plain feel good together?

Other possibilities:
jubilance, cheerfulness, elation, laughter, mirth.

3. The Fruit of the Spirit Is Peace.

Is there an increasing quiet in our hearts, in our home, in our love?

More and more are we truly content, relaxed?

More words for pondering:

serenity, composure, harmony, repose, tranquillity, stillness.

4. The Fruit of the Spirit Is Long-Suffering.

Is there an increasing stretch in our attitudes?

Do the little oddities in each other and in all others disturb us less?

Are we more patient? More even-tempered?

Jesus stood for something, and we will too. We do not want to become so broad that we flatten out into "anything goes." But even when we must disagree, can we do so with a greater appreciation of the other person's rights?

Also:

forbearance, flexibility, tolerance, adaptability.

5. The Fruit of the Spirit Is Gentleness.

Are we increasingly kind, more courteous, softer in our touch?

Physically, mentally, verbally, are we more tender?

Long-suffering deals with our attitude toward those things people do to us. Gentleness asks the opposite: are we more Christ-like in the things we do to other people?

Added possibilities:

docile, soothing, compassionate, mellow, gracious.

6. The Fruit of the Spirit Is Meekness.

Is there a growing self-honesty in each of us?

From the many interpretations of meekness, we have worked out our own definition: "True meekness is to know the difference between what we are right now and what God intends us to be."

For us, closing these gaps is one more achievement toward which great marriages move. "Measure us, Lord. Keep measuring us."

Supplementary words:
mildness, humility, yielding, resignation, submission.

7. *The Fruit of the Spirit Is Goodness.*
More and more do we seek to be a blessing?
Do we reach out to help, make an effort to do something good, say something kind, lift another?

There is a goodness that counts itself good because it isn't bad. But Christian goodness is never inert. It doesn't hold back in the face of need or hesitate to act for the welfare of another.

More words for thinking:
ministry, helpfulness, generosity, service.

8. *The Fruit of the Spirit Is Faith.*
These fears of ours, are they on the decline?
Do we worry less, trust more?

Do we really believe there is a power greater than our own?

When we are anxious, are we better able to share our anxieties with each other and trust the Lord?

Additional possibilities:
reliance, belief, confidence, assurance.

9. *The Fruit of the Spirit Is Temperance.*
Are we more and more in charge of our emotions?
Are we growing in that self-control which is truly control by Christ?

The Bible says, "In him all things hold together" (Col. 1:17, RSV).

If the Spirit of the Lord is really at work in us, we should rattle less, scatter less, explode less. Is this how it is with us?

Temperance also reflects these traits:
self-restraint, self-rule, self-mastery, self-discipline.

Anyone pondering these questions in depth will realize this truth: there are no graduates from the school of the soul. No degrees, no diplomas.

Love, joy, peace,
   long-suffering, gentleness, goodness,
      faith, meekness, temperance
         are not accomplishments.
These are lifetime goals.

Or won't it be even better if they are part of our heavenly pilgrimage, too? That will keep us busy well into eternity, won't it? Maybe forever?

Lips never err, when wisdom keeps
the door.

Old saying

━━━━━━━━

Thus Saith the Lord

Martha was a lover of peace. That would be natural for
anyone who spent so much time with the Prince of Peace. But
her life as a lover of peace had some interesting variations.

For instance, if her children were arguing, fussing, she
would sometimes disappear. I did not like her leaving their
quarrels to me. So because I didn't like it we discussed it. (See
"Seven Official Rules for a Good, Clean Fight.") After we
discussed it, I liked her disappearances. Why? Because she
explained that she was doing her fade-away sometimes to pray.

I realized at once how right this was. Amazing how many
times the quarreling ended before she returned to the battle
zone. From her prayer chamber came peace.

There are those who would label this practice a clever
psychological maneuver. "They quit fussing when you take
away their audience." Yet for her it was far more than a
maneuver. For her it was a matter of "taking it to the Lord
in prayer." He loved children. He would know how to
reach them.

Sometimes she would do the same thing in public—public
quarrels, heated group conflicts, potential blowups of several
people, or of many. In every one of these situations I've seen
her quietly praying.

Sometimes she did more than pray. This was one of those times. I wasn't there, but I heard the report. Many, many times I heard it, and every time it was exciting. It came from a Sunday school class, the first adult class in our new Houston church. This was one of the first Sundays too, so it was new to everyone.

Organizing a new church is exciting, but it also has its hazards. One hazard is the gathering together of maneuvering hopers. What are they hoping for? They are hoping to take over. They come from near or far, and how fortunate can we be? They have arrived to mold this new work their way. Watch them now. They will tell you immediately they are on the Lord's side. Then if you listen closely you can tell whose side the Lord is on.

Slowly, sometimes not so slowly, they work their way into places of authority. Any place where they can dominate will do. And if they cannot dominate they may go away. If they do dominate, the others may go away.

On that first Sunday in our new church school the adult teacher was indeed the dominant type, a handsome man, all smiles, holding forth on his chosen theme: "All the Jews Are Going to Hell." It was largely his own curriculum, well fortified with proof-texts and quotes from leading authorities who thought exactly as he thought. He spoke with enthusiasm, with vigor, giving his theme the business—and giving all Jews the business too.

Ten minutes before the closing bell a young woman stood, waited for the teacher to breathe, then asked for the floor. In her deep and quiet voice she began: "I've been listening to every word you've said, sir, and I want you to know I couldn't disagree more.

"Have you ever noticed that the Lord we worship never, not once, ever told anyone they were going to hell? Never an individual, never a group, certainly never a race. Yes, He said, 'Ye are in danger of hellfire' but that's as close as He ever came to anything like the sweeping statements you've been making.

"I for one am offended by this presentation. How does anyone know what contact the Lord has with anyone at the time of death? Who are *we* to assign blocks of people to their eternal home? God is the judge of all. The Bible tells us clearly that we are all sinners. But that is not the good news. The good news is that *all* are welcome in the Father's house. He will not turn any away. Salvation is *His* to extend anywhere, to anyone, anytime.

"Perhaps now I should introduce myself. I am a member of this new church, and I am particularly fond of our new pastor. I like the way he thinks, and I can tell you for sure he wouldn't approve this lesson either. My name is Martha, and I am the new pastor's wife. Thank you."

=====

I wish I had been in the class that day. Those who were there said it was among the finest things they'd ever heard. One visitor from England said, "The lady was absolutely smashing!"

Was anyone turned off by what she said? I'm sure some were, but I'm also sure of this: for everyone turned off, there were many more turned on.

Most of them, I think, would have liked it for this one reason: it is a very good work to defend the absent who are being attacked.

Amazing defender, Martha. So shy as a child, so timid as a teenager, so preferring the background as an adult. Yet now and then when she felt a holy urge, there she was, standing to defend someone. Or rising even to defend a whole people. There she was coming out of her seat to say, clearly, definitely, unequivocably,

"Thus saith the Lord!"

She knew that the weaker sex was really
the stronger sex because of the weakness
of the stronger sex for the weaker sex.

Anonymous

The Submissive Wife, Oh?

If you had heard Martha give a talk, you'd have thought,
"This lady is a natural speaker." But she wasn't. Actually she
did not begin her speaking career until the later years of her
life. And Martha's transformation from quiet observer to
smooth performer was a complete surprise. It was to me, and
it was to those who knew her in both roles.

Van and Treva Jane were two of our best friends ever. Best
best friends describes it for Martha and Treva Jane. They were
also prayer partners. All this was years before, during our
Oklahoma pastorate. Because Van was an international oil
executive, they moved often to places far away like England,
Argentina, Libya. So Treva Jane and Martha could soon be
friends only by mail, prayer partners at a distance. On retirement, Van and Treva Jane moved to California.

Some years after their move we held a workshop in Palm
Springs. Treva Jane and Van attended, and it was one grand
reunion for us.

In a recent letter Treva Jane describes their reaction. "Martha's gift for loving unconditionally not only worked magic
when applied to you, Charlie, it also taught you to use the
same approach, so that you were able to love Martha from her
original shyness into the self-confident, poised woman who
could participate smoothly with you in your workshops and

on national TV. Remembering the painfully shy young woman who moved to Ponca City, Oklahoma, so many years ago, it was hard to recognize the self-assured Martha who took part in the workshop we attended in Palm Springs."

She overcredits me, because the truth was somewhat different. It actually happened one day when I was speaking at a large husband-wife conference in a southern state. Martha was with me.

———

A Russian philosopher proposes the following theory: Sometimes people are dramatically vaulted out of the crowd to a higher level. Suddenly comes an impetus. Just as suddenly an inspired someone responds. Leaving the plateau, as though by one giant leap, upward they go and life for them is never the same again.

Something like that happened to Martha at this conference. The impetus came from a clergyman to whom I shall forever be grateful. I had been speaking on family life, marriage, parenting. This session's particular emphasis was time commitments, scheduling, family togetherness. When I had finished, a confident-looking pastor stood for rebuttal.

"I do not doubt your enthusiasm," he began, "but I seriously question your reporting. One evening each week for your wife? Another night the same week for family night? Five children? Each child every month one night out with Dad? I cannot believe it. I too pastor a large congregation. If you're as successful as I assume you are, there is simply no way you could spare that much time. Are you sure you're not telling us how you'd *like* it to be?"

In a flash, there she was at the podium. "I rise to inform you, sir," she began, "my husband is telling you exactly the way it is." Then with the tongue of a polished orator she held those six hundred listeners spellbound.

Methodically, inspirationally, she made her points.

- The more people who come to us for loving, the more we need time for regular loving in our own little cluster, plus one-on-one.
- The best ministry possible to families in our church is a loving ministry to our own family.
- That pastor who puts his wife first witnesses, as he could in no other way, to marriages crying for direction.

On and on she went, bringing tears to the eyes of thankful wives, making them laugh, making them think, making believers, making her points, heralding her pastor-husband.

When she had finished, as one body they rose to give her a standing ovation.

That night when we returned to our room I held her close and thanked her.

"Charlie," she said, "you mean they've been *paying* you for this? I never knew it could be so much fun. Let's do it again."

So we did, again and again. Certainly she worked at it, honed her newfound skills, polished her performance. But from that moment she was on her way to becoming one superb public speaker.

═════

Some themes are like an old dog. Most of the time they lie around the yard sleeping; then someone whistles, and they get up to bark a few times. But when nothing significant happens, they hunker down again, awaiting another whistle.

"The Submissive Wife" was such a theme, and it was not one of Martha's favorites. Yet in every workshop here they came again—questions, questions, same old questions: "What do you think of Ephesians 5:22?" "Should a wife always be the one to give in?" "When is it all right to say, 'No. I've got to be me'?"

Finally Martha decided she would prepare a talk. She would study every biblical reference on the theme. She'd listen, discuss, think, pray, and then have her say. "The Submissive Wife, Oh?" was her title. And these were her thoughts—notes from which she spoke.

═══════

"An obscure translation of Ephesians 5:22 says, 'You wives must willingly obey your men in everything.' Can you accept that as it stands? I can't, and it sounds like a man, doesn't it? It was. Do you suppose he was married?

"Colossians 3:19 gives this advice for husbands: 'Married men, be affectionate to your wives and never treat them harshly.' I tell Charlie if he'll live by Colossians, I'll live by Ephesians.

"Making the Bible say what we want it to say is dangerous. But so is taking texts out of context. That's where I believe the submissive wife theme makes for confusion.

"So I decided to research the subject. I asked myself three questions: What does the whole Bible say? What does it say that is often overlooked? What does it say to me personally?

"Here is one thing the Bible says before it tells women to submit. Ephesians 5:21, speaking to both husbands and wives, gives this opening directive, 'Submit yourselves to each other.'

"Now that makes more sense. Does your husband have days when he isn't thinking straight? Charlie does. On days like this I tell him, 'You're not up to your usual brilliance. Go to your workshop. Build something.' What does he do? He thanks me and goes. Then on the rare days when I'm not up to par he does the same for me. We heartily recommend some well-worked-out agreement on two-way submission.

"What does the word 'submit' really mean? Scholars disagree, but one meaning comes through clearly. This is our lovely English word 'yield.'

"Let's consider. When should a wife yield? When should I yield?

> I decided I should yield when it doesn't really matter.
>
> I should yield when it matters more to Charlie than it matters to me.
>
> I should yield when I'm wrong.

"You won't tell your husband, but when I did some checking, guess what? If I yield always on these *three* occasions, it's amazing—the scale tips very heavy on Charlie's side. Now you already know where I'm heading, don't you? You try it. If you yield that much to your husband, how could he possibly refuse to yield when it really does matter to you?

"Always, then, twenty-one comes before twenty-two. So here it is straight from 5:21, 'Submit yourselves to each other.'

"This second often-forgotten truth behind biblical yielding has to be the final answer: *We are to yield together to the Lord.*

"Where does it say that? One of the New Testament's most pensive chapters on married love is 1 Peter 3. Here we find some of the Bible's most specific directives for marriage at its best.

"Invite your husband to study it with you. You'll be glad you did, and so will he. Here you will learn the art of soul-to-soul living with the Lord. But that's not all. You will also discover the pure-gold reason why any couple should yield together. 'Do this,' the writer says, 'so that nothing will interfere with your prayers.'

"Now that really is some reason for yielding, isn't it?"

TOGETHER

Give not that which is holy unto the
dogs.

Matthew 7:6, KJV

Bongo of the Congo

Martha loved dogs, and we had many for her to love. At
one time early in our marriage we owned a sizable kennel of
collies. "Hallelujah" was our kennel name, and our entries bore
their title proudly in the show ring, especially "Hallelujah
Buz." We named our dogs, as we did our cats, for biblical
characters. (See Gen. 22:21; 1 Chron. 5:14; Jer. 25:23.)

We had fun with our collies. We met some real people
characters at shows and visiting other kennels. We also learned
much about the animal kingdom, but finally we gave it up for
a good reason.

We were doing what the Bible told us not to do. We were
giving too much time, too much energy, too much thought,
to the dogs. Now and then this question even crossed our
minds: Were we ourselves getting a bit doggy?

From that time on we never owned another collie. Other
breeds, yes, and what an assortment: Samson, the Saint Ber-
nard; Shadrack, the Airedale; Prudence, the miniature schnau-
zer; Snowplow and Blizzard, pure white Great Pyrenees; and
Smitty, Granny, and Winston (non-biblical names for those
who arrived already named). Martha loved them all, with a
special love for each.

Then came Bongo of the Congo. Bongo was a pedigreed, registered, blue-blooded basenji, the barkless dog of Africa, medium-sized, brown-and-white, with curly tail, pointed ears, and deep worry wrinkles on the brow. "Super personality, great pet, bundles of fun." That's what the ads said.

But Bongo was none of these, unless super personality might mean super ugly all the way. Yet he was very dependable. Every day without fail he would bite someone!

He also had a howl, a howl so loud it many times made up for the barks he couldn't bark. His favorite howling time was anywhere between midnight and six in the morning, of which serenading our next-door neighbor took a dim view. Not to be outdone, she opened her window and howled back! Who could blame her? It was very effective. Not quite as loud, not quite as rhythmical, not quite as long as a howl from Bongo, yet almost. It was competition enough between them, to utterly wreck the sleep of an entire neighborhood.

Bongo had another fault. He ran away regularly. Unfortunately (for us) this was too small a town. We all knew each other rather well. We also knew each other's dogs. So after one night of howling elsewhere, Bongo was brought back to howl again for us.

Martha finally put an end to this fiasco. God bless her soul, she had her limit, and this was the limit. "Now hear this," she began. (I always listened up fast when she began "Now hear this.") "Remember the first day Bongo bit your hand when you took him from the crate? From that day I have not liked Bongo. Believe me, I've tried. I've prayed for him, for me, for you, for the neighbors, for the next one he bites. I have even prayed for the people who sold him to us. And do you know what I get when I pray these prayers? I get it on highest authority, Charlie. *The Lord does not expect us to neaten up the whole world. From some things, praise God, He exempts us.* That's how it is, with this disastrous character. Bongo has got to go!"

She was right. Once more we were giving that which was holy unto dogs, so Bongo went. Where he went was to a long, long lane out in the country. We gave him, his collar, pedigree, dog dishes, the food we hadn't fed him yet—everything—to a nice old, frightened couple way out there. They wanted a dog that would bite people.

How did he do? Just fine, thank you. We saw them now and then on Saturdays when the citizenry would come to town for groceries. No exception, superb reports. Fact is, they said, he'd probably made it possible for them to stay on the home place longer than they could ever have stayed without him. They liked him. They loved him. And did he ever love what he had been called to do—bite, howl, keep predators away.

Isn't that a nice ending to what, for us, was a horrible experience?

In the Book of Ecclesiastes there is a verse which says, "To everything there is a season and a purpose to everything under the sun."

Including Bongo?
Yes,
including Bongo!

Understand, it was forty-odd years ago when I heard this passionate Bongo address from Martha. Certainly some of the original phrases, particular words may have dimmed a bit, but not much. When Martha's ire reached maximum, both content and delivery reached maximum too. And always right then I admired her, respected her, registered what she said, and loved her with a special love.

One thing I do know for sure: her liberating phrase from that original speech has never dimmed and never will. For us together it became kind of a life motto, a support, an emancipator. How many times did one of us say it to the other, or both of us say it together? And how many times did it bless us? Many, many.

> The good Lord doesn't expect us
> to neaten up the whole world.
> From some things,
> praise God,
> He exempts us.

These are but the outskirts of his ways;
and how small a whisper do we hear
of him!

Job 26:14, RSV

Whispers of His Love

Mysterious happenings are a part of nearly every life—
sometimes bothersome, sometimes devastating, sometimes
blessings in disguise, but almost always puzzling.

Some observers lump all of life's unusual events under one
heading: ESP, extrasensory perception. Good for a lively discussion, fun for party games, but not much more. Perhaps that
is a tidy way to deal with what's not understandable: give it
a name and dismiss it.

Yet by any other moniker these unexplained events do
leave us wondering. Call them odd, eerie, bizarre, far out, or
plain coincidence, something is going on. Behind the scenes,
a touch of the divine maybe? Good happenings from a good
angel? Bad happenings from an angel turned bad? Or wouldn't
it be exciting if there really was something, some One out
there with a special interest in me? In us? In our goings-on?

After we started praying together, Martha and I began to
feel some things we'd never felt before. Sometimes strange
blendings of events, people coming together unexpectedly, old
problems solved. Maybe an unseen hand would be touching
us, nudging, moving us forward, holding us back. Perhaps an
inner voice prompting us to go, come, stay, say this, do not
say that.

Mostly these were good times, sometimes very, very good. Scary now and then, very scary, but all much too real for light dismissal.

Often we were left awed, and almost always we discussed what was happening. Then we prayed and praised God for what to us were brushes of the angels' wings. So very real, incomprehensible most of the time, but highly authentic.

The story you are about to hear is true, proven, an event couched every way in love. Couched in love reaching across continents, love impossible to fully understand. But for the four of us who were there, it was more clearly understandable in this beautiful definition of Job, "These are but the outskirts of His ways; and how small a whisper do we hear of Him."

<hr>

Wolfsburg, Germany, is an exciting city. The city of Volkswagens—five thousand daily. The Scripture says, "Let everything be done decently and in order." That's how they do it in Wolfsburg. System. Smooth.

We had come to Wolfsburg to buy a Volkswagen for our high-school son. This was Peter's graduation present, pre-ordered and everything exactly the way he wanted it. Color right. Accessories right. And oh, that Volkswagen welcome to Wolfsburg!

We stayed in one of those spotless German *pensions*— feather beds, plus breakfast, at bargain rates.

It was here I dreamed an unusual dream. I don't dream much, just enough to keep it interesting, and pleasant themes usually, in color. I have a friend who is big on interpreting dreams. I'm not. I've always thought of mine as a nice bonus to an already fun life.

This one was about Grandma. My mother-in-law was extra special. She liked me too. What I liked most about her were the reflections of God I saw in her. Having already given me her daughter, she did another fine thing. She kept giving me the feeling that life with the Lord was 100 percent natural.

I should tell you here that Wolfsburg was only one stop in a thirty-day tour of Europe, including the Scandinavian countries.

It was Wednesday, July 21. In my dream we had arrived in Copenhagen, and there was a message. Grandma had died, and we must return to the States. The most vivid part of my dream was Peter in his little Volkswagen. It seemed to weave its way in and out of the dream, past the red cows and white barns, through the little towns, up and down the pleasant hills of Denmark and Germany, then to Amsterdam for return shipment.

The next morning I told the dream to Martha. Sometime back we had agreed to tell each other our dreams. And was I ever glad I'd told her this one!

That night at dinner in Hamburg I felt the nudge to share it with our boys. Timothy, our youngest, didn't like it. But with the typical "wisdom" of parenthood, we assured him it was only a dream. It took Peter, with the greater wisdom of youth, to say, "But Tim, Grandma is eighty-one. Let's face it. She's going to die sometime." So each of us put it on the shelf with things to be forgotten.

Friday we had a fascinating time in Grandma's hometown. At twenty-one she had come from Odense, Denmark, to the Midwest and Iowa. We had dinner with her relatives, visited St. Knud's Church where she had been baptized, and looked for the homes where she had grown up. They were still there, in excellent shape. Her father had been a carpenter.

Saturday we arrived in Copenhagen and reported to our travel agent. We had put the dream away, but not very far.

On our arrival at the hotel, Tim headed for the desk. The rest of us stood in line to cash some checks. There are some moments to be remembered forever. One of mine came when Tim handed me this note:

"Important. Call Mr. Petersen, Portland, Oregon, immediately." Then his number, and that was all.

Mr. Petersen is my brother-in-law. We looked at each other without a word. We went to our room, placed the call, and it was exactly as we knew it would be.

"Charlie, I'm sorry to tell you that Mom died this morning. Pastor Tange said she ate a hearty breakfast, then went to her room, and died. Wasn't that just like Mom?"

It was. For a long time we sat there blending our feelings. We cried. We prayed. Especially we thanked God for three days of preparation by way of "our" dream.

Three of us took off the next morning on a return flight. You can believe it was an intense moment as we watched our eighteen-year-old drive away in his Volkswagen. Of course, he made it safely past the red cows and white barns, through the little towns, and over the gentle hills to Amsterdam. Then on he went to Iowa for the funeral. Eighteen-year-olds can do so much more than we as parents are prone to believe. I tell you this because Martha had said, "Shouldn't one of us go with Peter?" To which he observed, like the philosopher he is, "Mom, I'll do anything to make you feel better. If you want Dad to go with me, that's fine. But wouldn't it spoil the dream?"

They have the nicest custom at Grandma's church. After the funeral, everyone comes together in the parlor for coffee, which for Danish people also means sandwiches of infinite variety, cookies of infinite variety, cakes of infinite variety, conversation of infinite variety.

I found myself talking with some of Grandma's friends. What I learned was that she had been worried about our itinerary. We had asked our travel agent to send it to each member of our family, but she hadn't received her copy. Someone down the line had directed it to the wrong town. We knew this because it arrived two days after her death.

"Do you suppose," one of her friends said, "that she told the Lord to get in touch with you? She hadn't been feeling quite up to par. I wonder if she sensed something?"

"You don't think that's impossible, do you?" That's how Bertel answered. Bertel and his wife were two of Grandma's favorites. They took her to church on Sunday. "I don't think that's any harder to believe than your dreaming it before it happened," he said. "In fact, knowing Marie and how she lived with the Lord, I think that's exactly what happened. She told Him to look you up, and He did."

There is one other small part I haven't told you. On the day we left home, Martha wrote her brother a note. That was very unusual. They had the best of feelings for each other, but they also had one of those relationships for which that's enough. They did have great times when they were together, but other than that, they let it go and loved each other in silence. Yet for some reason she felt compelled that day to send him this message: "We will be at Five Swans Hotel in Copenhagen on July 24."

There were nineteen known stops on our thirty-day schedule. These were confirmed reservations. The rest were of the do-it-yourself variety. In the three days prior to Grandma's death, we were free-floating through Germany and Denmark. The day following we were to board ship for three days' incommunicado sailing along the coasts of Sweden and Norway.

Why had she died that particular day? For what reason had Martha selected that particular stop to tell her brother? Why had we been given three days' notice by the dream? What is the explanation? How do we solve these mysteries?

Again we must go to the Book of Job and his lovely line "how small a whisper do we hear of him!"

This has to be where the answer is. God in His love cares about us. He knows what we need to know. He knows where we need to be. It is not ours to push or crowd or hurry. Ours is to respond and follow His lead, and listen for His whispers.

As I have said, when we began praying together, mysterious things began to happen in our love, great and wonderful things. The more we prayed, the more they happened. And the more they happened, the more we knew for sure there is between human and divine a real connection—if we stay tuned!

In Christ there is no east or west,
In him no south or north;
But one great fellowship of love
Throughout the whole wide earth.

John Oxenham

Love in Full Extension

Martha had a missionary aunt in China. Aunt Anna was an imposing woman, large of stature, strong of voice, promoter par excellence. Always somewhat pushy. And when it came to mission candidates, Aunt Anna was very, very pushy.

Whenever Aunt Anna came home on furlough, Martha got the full treatment. "You, little girl, would make a fine missionary to China. Let me describe the exciting life you'd lead." Etcetera on forever.

Junior High, same battle, next skirmish.

Senior High, ditto.

College, now Aunt Anna called up the troops. "Just think how the Lord could use you in China with that home economics major."

You will sense that my reporting here may be somewhat biased. Aunt Anna did not take kindly to me! Even the casual observer could sense it. To her, I was the villain, come to purloin her prize-catch future missionary for China. But for me this was always compensated by another fact. To Martha I was the hero come to save her. "Charlie," she would purr, "you kept me from going to China, but you also saved me from Aunt Anna. Thank you."

Yet behind her smile when she said it was an ever-present interest in missions, which, of course, would be a natural for Martha. If she and the Lord were friends from the inside out, of course she would care about all God's children. She would care about all his adults too, in China and elsewhere.

This was the Martha spirit straight from the Lord. He said He would not be satisfied until the whole world belonged to Him. We, His people, have no choice. We must pray, plan, and give what we can. In every way we must love in full extension.

═════

Being leaders of a church which gave fifty-fifty (a dollar for us, a dollar for others), we couldn't be blind to this question: Does the Lord want *us* to match *our* dollars in the same way?

He did! From the first small checks of our marriage we lived by this formula:

give ten percent;

save ten percent;

spend the rest with thanksgiving and praise.

No, it wasn't easy at first. It wasn't easy either sometimes as the years moved along. But running it through the blender of money memories, we knew this: very few decisions we ever made matched that formula for right moves. Out of it came countless good things: system, satisfaction, vision, but above all the blessings was growth that brought more blessings.

═════

Give a man a meal, and he thanks you. But though you have fed him, you have also humiliated him. Give him the means of supporting himself, and you have given him the greatest gift of all—dignity.

The Abundance Foundation is dedicated to agricultural missions. Established early in our career of writing and speaking, it has had a fascinating history. Water buffalo and goats in the Philippines, feeding the hungry, providing milk and meat. Chickens and pigs at a leper colony in Korea. Mules in Thailand. Dairy herds in Zaire. Rabbits in Nigeria. Other projects in Haiti, Ghana, Gambia, India.

Cattle, chickens, pigs, honeybees, riding horses, machinery, and buildings at a farming school for retarded youngsters in Virginia.

David runs a peanut combine at that school. Much too often the retarded are told, "You can't. You'll never be able to." That's what David heard.

"Before I came here," he said, "they told me I could never do nothin'. Now look. I'm running the tractor. Next month I go to work for a farmer. That's pretty neat, don't you think?"

When he put his arms around us to thank us, Martha and I did think it was pretty neat.

It is neat, more than pretty neat, how God reaches out to touch His own. Prediction: Those who will make a specific commitment for giving, saving, spending will one day discover for themselves just how neat it is.

I have a feeling too about Aunt Anna these days. All the prod and promo of one pushy aunt wasn't wasted. Martha, with her zeal for missions, did get the message. So here's a belated word of commendation for you, Aunt Anna. Thanks for a missionary wife. She's pretty neat, don't you think?

In her tongue is the law of kindness.
Proverbs 31:26, KJV

Incident at the Garage Door

Have you ever backed your car out of the garage without opening that main door?

If you have, you know there is no other feeling quite like it. Crash—smash—utter devastation. And if it should be the kind with glass windows—glass, glass everywhere. Yet even the sound of all this wreckage is minor compared to the question you are asking, "How could I be so stupid?"

Was your mate watching? If not, did she come rushing from the house to see if a truck had run amok?

What did she say? Comes now a moment for some special bonding—or otherwise.

The first time I did it (my record is two), Martha was standing by the kitchen door to wave good-bye. Why didn't she signal me to stop? No time. I was looking at the gas gauge. Repeat: crash—smash—utter devastation. Then that sinking sensation, "How could I be so stupid?"

Now here is Martha by my side:

"Are you hurt, Charlie? I'm so, so sorry. But don't you feel bad. Remember, I love you. I've come close myself to backing through that door. I was lucky. Let's go to work. I'll sweep up the glass; you take out the bolts. We'll undo it together, haul it to the dump, get it out of sight. Stop punishing yourself. Remember some of the dumb things I've done?"

I remembered. How could I ever forget the maiden flight of her pressure cooker lid? It was a new pressure cooker, and Martha was making one of her super, super stews. But somehow, she said later, she didn't have the lid on right. I was back in the study when suddenly, from the general vicinity of the kitchen, came a sonic boom.

Dashing to the rescue, I could see what had happened. Pressure cooker lid blown off, stew blown high. Stew, stew everywhere. Stew all over the maker of the stew. Stew all over the kitchen floor, refrigerator, stove, cabinets. Have you ever seen carrots, potatoes, beef, plus sundry other stew ingredients, imbedded in the ceiling?

Now what should a husband do at a pivotal moment like this?

Should he be a comedian? "Way to go, baby! You've been wanting to redo the kitchen. What imagination! Super start!"

Should he play judge? "How could you be so . . . ?" (Excellent control, there, Buster. Good moment to cease and desist.)

Or, taking a page from one loving wife and a garage door incident, should he say, "Put your head on my shoulder, darling. Cry a little. Let's praise the Lord you weren't killed by a flying lid. Don't punish yourself. That could happen to anyone. Remember the time I [*select any two*]."

Looking back on our forty-eight years, I wish I had always been the wisest of loving husbands. Some moments of our emergencies I'd like to have back. Why does it take so much time to learn the secret?

Most of us can work our way through to what we should say if we have time. But in those smash, crash, devastating moments when a marriage bonds or rifts a little, what then?

Wouldn't it be ever so fine to always have the right word for every emergency? Can we? Probably not by planning, or even by rehearsal, but by being tuned to the Inner Presence, we can.

Didn't our Lord say if we are in touch with His spirit, it would be given to us in crucial moments what to say?

This too was the Martha blessing: automatic kindness straight from the Source. That is a great quality in a person responding to big mistakes and little. It is also second to none for dumb mistakes like my backing the car through our garage door . . . closed.

========

"Go Where the Joy Is"

In Old Testament days, countries conquering countries made a familiar story. Plunder was common, and the spoils of war included capable people. Artisans, craftsmen, skilled workers of all kinds, teachers, and thinkers were prime booty. So were the movers and shakers, leaders and doers.

One translator, in plain, unvarnished language, tells it like it is. "The poor who have nothing" are to be left behind. The "so-called better class" will be carried away for service in Babylon (Jer. 39:9–10, AMP).

Usually when the conquering warriors came, they had been preceded by spies. Check the terrain; count the local troops; but one thing more: mark the "so-called better class" for capture. Locked up before the slaughter, these would be protected from the heat of battle. Then when the war was over they could be exported in good condition.

So Jeremiah was in prison, and we can be sure he was talking to the Lord. For his nation, for his friends, for his own future, he would be praying.

========

Martha and I had reached a time in our lives when we were praying about our future. We were in an exciting church.

People, people, everywhere. Challenge. Drama. Prestige. But we were also writing, conducting workshops, doing other exciting things away from home.

Writing and all that comes with it requires time. It also takes energy. Pastoring a large church demands time and energy too. So this double career had brought us to a crossroads.

A small island church off the coast of Georgia had extended us their invitation. Accepting would give us a church family plus writing time. Yet the pressure to remain where we were never let up.

What should we do?

Often in our Bible study, Martha would say, "Charlie, I think I've found something just for us." This time it came from Jeremiah: "Now I am taking the chains off your wrists and setting you free. If you want to go to Babylonia with me, you may do so, and I will take care of you. But if you don't want to go, you don't have to. You have the whole country to choose from, and you may go wherever you wish" (Jer. 40:4, GNB).

"Doesn't Jeremiah's problem touch on our problem?" she asked. "He's faced with a choice too. Should he go to Babylon and minister where the leaders are? Or should he stay and help the beaten folks at home?

"Listen to this last line again, 'You have the whole country to choose from, and you may go wherever you wish!' Do you get what I get from that? Isn't the Lord saying, 'Loosen up. If you stay, I'll find some other workers up there. If you go, I'll handle things here. You decide'?

"Of course, this kind of thinking could be dangerous. As I read the whole of Jeremiah, it wasn't always this way for him. There were times when the Lord wanted him to do what he didn't want to do. We've been there too, haven't we?

"But isn't this a wonderful fact? Sometimes the divine guidance seems to say, 'I gave you your mind, your feelings, your judgment. So now use what I gave you. I'm leaving it up to you. Either way you choose would please me. This time do what pleases you.'"

End of Martha's statement, except for one more phrase. Every couple from their serious Bible study together will have this experience. Suddenly, they come on these days of high visibility. They see now the meaning of things they had only seen on the surface before. The ambiguous becomes plain, and whispers of doubt change to songs of gladness.

This time it was like that for us. Straight from Jeremiah's answered prayer to an answer for us came these five words:

"Go where the joy is!"

And we went.

Some people seem forever locked in the status quo. Others tend invariably to flutter and excitement. Then there are those with another trait, exactly the right mix of old and new: conservative enough to never let go of eternal values, experimental enough to welcome fresh insight.

Martha was richly blessed with these qualities. Here is a quotation which she recorded in one of our notebooks. I know only two things about its source. It came from a novel she was reading, and the words are those of an old grandmother under fire for dabbling in the unfamiliar. "Land sakes, how's a body going to learn if we put up fences around all kinds of subjects and won't let our brains graze in 'em some?"

Risky? Not for Martha. With her base of a solid divine relationship, it would always be safe for her to graze around. And from that same base she could say, for our indecision, "If God is our dwelling place, does it matter all that much where we live?"

> Be ye angry, and sin not.
>
> *Ephesians 4:26, KJV*

═══════

The Lioness

Every good woman has many names. Every good woman deserves good titles too. One of mine for Martha was "Lioness." I named her that first when I came home for dinner one night and she met me dish in hand. The dish was carefully covered but not too carefully. From it, one of my favorite aromas.

"We are going," she said, "to see Oliver and Edna. Don't argue. Just come along." Whenever she gave me that look, I did not argue. I just went along.

"What's in the pan?"

"Pecan rolls."

"Lucky Oliver and Edna. Nobody makes pecan rolls like your pecan rolls."

So off we went.

Oliver and Edna were active members of our church. Somewhat elderly and nice folks except for one thing: they never entertained an unexpressed thought. These two were what the professionals call "heavy vocalizers."

Recently they had been more negative than usual, and the reason was my new book, *The Stork Is Dead.* Written for the young, it came out of a "Sex and Dating" column I'd been doing for *Teen* magazine. It would be natural that an older generation might misunderstand. The book was not written for the older generation. And it certainly was not written for Oliver and Edna.

They weren't the only members of our church who found their minister a bit embarrassing right now. Others had fueled the conversational bonfires too, but Martha knew something I didn't know. We were bearing rolls for the ringleaders, and they had an extensive following.

They met us at the door with their usual Oliver and Edna welcome—hearty, warm. They really were a fun pair most of the time, but not right now for the pastor's wife.

One thing Martha could never handle with equilibrium was criticism of her Charlie. Oliver and Edna had gone too far. Martha was about to apply the ax to the roots of this particular "fiasco" (her word).

Actually, I'd heard very little about the things people were saying. I'd been on the road promoting the book. Then too, authors know they'll meet with variant reactions; they also know that can be a good thing. The agents say that almost any kind of talk, good or bad, will help sell books.

"I baked you some pecan rolls," my defender began, and that brought the usual positive reaction. Her rolls were well known from our church dinners.

Then, when the "up" notes had subsided, she went on: "It has come to my attention that you have been criticizing Charlie. We have a rule, Charlie and I, that we will not tell a secret, or bother ourselves with public complaint, until we've heard it at least five times. Well, your five times have arrived, and I came here to tell you that you are going to *shut up!* The things you are saying can't be good for the church, and they most certainly aren't good for me. From now on, then, when you're about to criticize my husband, you will remember my rolls and how they came to you. Understand?"

They understood. Of course there were the usual protestations, "Martha dear, you must have been misinformed. Where did you hear all this? Who told you?"

"I have been misinformed?" she questioned. "Well, that *is* good news. Now we can continue friends as usual."

Then we left, and on the way home I took her hand. I noticed her hand was shaking. Of course she would be shaking! Leaving our normal character to do what we know needs doing can be a bit scary.

That night at dinner I told her how proud I was of her, how satisfying it is to live with someone who loves that much.

She smiled, served me another pecan roll, and queried, "Charlie, exactly how angry do you think the Lord was when He drove those money changers from the temple? It seems like such a fine line between enough and too much. How can we know for sure?"

"Well," I answered, "you weren't trying to drive anyone out. He was only trying to purify the temple. Isn't that all you were doing?"

Then, putting her arms around me, she said with a smile (her coy one), "Thank you, darling. I do so like your biblical interpretations. And you have noticed, haven't you, how much I like you?"

"Yes," I answered, "I have noticed."

Blessed is the man
who is married to a woman
sometimes kitten, sometimes cat,
and sometimes at the right time,
pure lioness.

Fair is the white star of twilight
And the sky clearer
At the day's end;
But she is fairer.

Shoshone love song

What Did Martha Look Like?

It is almost impossible for words to capture true beauty, isn't it? But people often ask, "What did Martha look like?" For answer, I will tell a story, a true story. It happened several years ago when we were living at Fripp Island, South Carolina. Charming spot, twenty miles out in the Atlantic. Miles and miles of white beach. Acres and acres of pine trees, golf courses, sand dunes, trails. But nothing was more fascinating than the sea, calm or otherwise. For beauty of the majestic kind, the sea takes top billing.

At Fripp Island very close in second place for beauty is the marsh. Changing color by the hour, reflecting the sun, picking up the cloud shades, variant in splendor. Even with no sun, no clouds, it's always interesting. Filled with secret sea life, of inestimable value to the ecology, these are the East Coast marshlands.

How do I know all this? I know because we lived on the marsh. High home, with kitchen and living room upstairs, a spacious deck from which on a clear day we could see forever. "There's Cuba to the south. New York up there to the right!" I'm kidding, you can be sure, but you get the idea. Ours was a distant view.

So what did Martha look like? This now, is what Martha looked like.

Homer and Eunice Larsen had come for a visit. They are among our very favorite people. Homer is now, and has been for years, pastor of Martha's home church in Cedar Falls, Iowa. Warm, loving, powerful, jolly, a jovial leader. And Eunice is the perfect mate for a man like Homer. Both are the kind of people you like to have come see you.

So there we sat on our front deck paying tribute to the colors, listening to the sounds of hidden sea life. Way out there was a glittering backdrop, the ocean. "Did you ever see anything more beautiful?" A likely question from our visitors.

That question led naturally now to another question. Especially with Homer and Eunice, the next question would come naturally: "What is the most beautiful view you have ever seen?"

Here are friends examining their memories for beauty:

"I think for pure grandeur I'd take the Swiss Alps, especially the view from Mount Pilatus."

"Something like the feeling you get in the Colorado Rockies, don't you think? We lived in Colorado for two years, and I never got tired of Longs Peak or Mount Meeker from our kitchen window."

"What about Denmark? The countryside, so soft, so soothing. Neat, neat farms, cows grazing. Plus Copenhagen. Ah, Copenhagen."

"Have you been to Alaska? The glaciers? Giant vegetables, giant flowers of many kinds."

A well-traveled group, obviously. Great listening, all three. But where was number four? "You sick, Charlie? Waiting to get a word in edgewise? Come on, tell us what you're thinking."

Then I told them what I was thinking. "I think you've all missed it. At least you have for me. For me the most beautiful sight in all God's creation is Martha.

Martha coming down the aisle on Sundays while I sit in my pulpit chair watching the worshipers gather.

Martha turning from her stove to smile at me when I tell her I like the aroma of her kitchen.

Martha stepping from her shower in the morning."

═════

For me she was "full of wisdom and perfect in beauty" (Ezekiel 28:12, KJV). Through my eyes, *that* is what Martha looked like.

MALIGNANT

Neither the sun nor death can be looked
at with a steady eye.

François

Dark Clouds Gathering

Long before Martha was diagnosed with cancer, I had seen
the shadows. Dark clouds were gathering in her sky, and in
mine. Off there in the distance, heavy clouds were shaping.
Sometimes when we sat together in the evening, there were
new lines around her eyes, a drawn look on her face.

Once when I came into the barn, she was bent over almost
doubled from exhaustion. She'd been using the weed-eater on
our ditches. Tidy she was in everything. Yard work for her
was like a day at the beach. Fun.

She especially liked cutting weeds, mowing, anything
with rhythm, anything that would show results. But now
here she was in the barn struggling for breath. I knew immediately something must be wrong. I knew she knew it too,
because she didn't hesitate when I suggested a quick trip to
the doctor.

"Notice anything unusual lately?" he began.

"Yes, sometimes in her sleep, her heartbeat seems too fast,"
I answered. "Breath too heavy. And one thing more. After a
good night she's still tired."

So now to a thorough examination, and the semi-good
news. "Nothing too serious. Must be your age. You're seventy

now. I think you're a normal seventy. Rest. Take it easy. Let's see how it goes."

How it went was not good. Breathing much too heavy, persistent tiredness. So back to the doctor for more examinations. New ones, the old ones again, all inconclusive.

Referrals next: lung specialist, heart specialist, neurologist, oncologist, radiologist. And then the news nobody wants to hear.

"Something shadowy on the lungs. Something we've got to understand before we go on. It's a real puzzler. You never smoked, you've never been exposed to the lung destroyers. Could be cancer, but before we can treat it, we must know for sure. That means we're down to one choice, exploratory surgery on the lungs."

He was a good specialist with superior credentials, but still, he could give us nothing definite. Next step, send the biopsies to Birmingham, Philadelphia, the Mayo Clinic. How long do we wait? Ten days? Two weeks?

In the meantime, "Would you feel better if we sent you somewhere? We think we know what it is, but someone else might find what we can't find. Anyone you say, anywhere. We'll send our findings. Think it over. Examine the options. You make the decision."

Together in our ministry we had seen hopeful parishioners off for Mexico, Austria, Sweden, the Orient. Other places too, other doctors in our own country. Yet almost no exception, they came home with heavy hearts. Some borrowed time maybe, but the end result was the same. So we prayed; we discussed; we prayed some more; and we opted to stay where we were. Good doctors, home, family, friends.

=====

The four most beautiful words in the English language are, "It is *not* malignant." But we were not to hear them.

Reports:

Birmingham: "Uncertain."
Philadelphia: "Uncertain."
Mayo Clinic: "Certain. Cancer.
    Widespread. Aggressive."

Cancer
    equals ominous, frightening, terror in the soul;
    equals despair, denial, anger;
    equals that exploratory operation
    to learn the type
        (needed for treatment),
    to learn the extent
        (needed to determine how
        much treatment).

═══

We stood by our car in the doctor's parking lot. We held each other close. The bird of our hope was down with a black bullet in its heart:

"Cancer. Widespread. Aggressive."

> May there be such a oneness between you
> in your marriage that when one of you
> weeps the other will taste salt.
>
> *Martin Buxbaum*

"Charlie, Are You All Right?"

No surgeon's knife had offended her body before, and to her it was a great offense. This day the doctors had gone into her lungs. Before they could begin treatment, they must have proof of cancer. And they found it. Extensive. Malignant. Bad news.

She'd been in the far-off places where postoperative patients go. She'd made hardly a movement, not even a flicker of those beautiful eyes. Total silence. Zero response.

Now it was eight and a half hours after her surgery. No one else was in the room, and I was holding her hand. Suddenly she awoke, looked at me, smiled, and said, "Charlie, are you all right?"

How does a person in great pain, pain of body, pain of soul, think first of others? Anyone can be gracious when success is sure and the skies are blue. But what will we do when the shadows come? Will we be able then to care about those around us? Can we put our own pain aside to know that others are hurting too?

Amazing grace, this kind of Divine otherness, and Martha had it in bountiful supply. All those years she had lived with the Inner Presence. Whatever she faced now, she would go on living His way.

Lord, I want to be like that. Each day, all day, and forever live in me. In good times and in bad, in life and in death, remind me that I was born to be a blessing. Make me a channel of Your grace.

(The Lord gave) beauty for ashes,
the oil of joy for mourning,
the garment of praise
for the spirit of heaviness.

Isaiah 61:3, KJV

Message in a Wig

We were driving to Atlanta for a wig. Wigs and chemo-therapy go together. Even at its kindest, chemo is a devastating treatment. And for a woman, one of its worst side effects is loss of hair.

She was silent most of the way, and that was unusual in the car. Both of us loved these driving times for talk, talk, talk.

As we approached the wig shop, she reached over and took my hand. "Charlie," she said, "do you know how awful this is for me? A woman's hair is her pride, her joy, something to create the many selves to match her many moods.

"I'm so downhearted, and I'm sorry too. I haven't talked much, but I've been praying, meditating. Would you like to know what happened? When I told the Lord how sad I am, He said, 'I understand. I know how you feel, and I'm sorry, because it really is a cross. But I have a suggestion. Why don't you think of me on my cross and imagine how lucky I would have felt to walk away with a wig!' "

So like Martha and her Lord—always the most intimate of conversations between them. The happy times she shared with Him, high moments they celebrated. Then in the lowest of her lows, always He had some special word for her; a note of encouragement straight from her Lord, with a touch of humor.

Her children rise up and call her blessed.
Proverbs 31:28, RSV

Karen

We have one daughter. Her name is Karen. She is a nurse, and she was an executive nurse with a clinical specialty in cancer. In this position, she ministered to the suffering. She held a young mother in her arms as the young mother died. She encouraged, loved, prayed with hurting families. She's that kind of girl.

Several years ago she came to her mother and me with a plan. She would like to quit her nursing job and go to law school. She would focus on health law, because there are so many legal needs in the health field. Nurses and doctors everywhere are looking for help. Hospitals are threatened by colossal problems these days. Suits, countersuits, all cry out for someone with medical knowledge and legal skills.

So she went into law. Three years she studied at the University of Georgia's fine law school. Then she joined the health law department of a major firm in Baltimore.

The church is not always in a building with steeple and stained glass. Sometimes the church emanates from the top-floor office of a city skyscraper.

When Karen requested a leave of absence to come and help care for her mother, the law firm agreed. Her background in the care of cancer patients made it seem right that she should be with her mother. With so many ways to keep in touch, she could continue working for the firm part-time. It was made plain that Karen would be welcome back full-time when she was ready to return.

Why would they do that?

Certainly she's a valuable member of the firm, and they hoped to keep her. For them her mix of law and medical background is invaluable. But isn't it always a special thrill when blessings come from unexpected places?

So she came, and she taught us how to think about cancer, how to talk about cancer. She showed us how to face facts and how to plan ahead. How to touch, how to encourage, how to change a bed with the patient on it—these things too she showed us. She explained care for the night and the daytime too. How to exercise the stubborn muscles, how to bandage, how to prepare food. All these. But was there any greater contribution than this? *She taught us how to face the fact of dying and how to deal with the act itself.*

So here's a special salute to all professionals in white coats, white caps, trained to minister with tender hands and tender hearts. But above all right now, a salute to those extra special angels who love with the extra special love required for cancer.

Surely there won't be cancer cases in heaven. But from watching one cancer nurse close up I'm absolutely sure of this:

there will be cancer nurses there
loving someone for the Lord,
someone whose need on arrival
is for extra love
and special care.

> To every thing there is a season, and
> a time to every purpose under the
> heaven . . . a time to keep silence, and a
> time to speak.
>
> *Ecclesiastes 3:1, 7, KJV*

"Let's Talk About Heaven"

Wheelchairs are a plus for those who need them. But for those who have always walked with grace, as Martha walked, the wheelchair is a chariot of wrath. No flowing now like a lovely stream, no more standing with dignity. Degrading.

Now the cancer goes to her spinal cord, and her legs simply will not move. Beautiful legs, shapely legs, almost gone, options down to one: the wheelchair.

What can we do? We can make the best of it, and we did. On days when she was up to a trip, we'd go riding. We had always loved our long rides, and all during our marriage they'd been like mini-retreats for us.

The Georgia mountains are so much fun for riding. Quaint little towns, festivals and fairs, antique shops, junk shops, sandwich shops. Interesting people, the natives. Interesting, too, the tourists.

At first she had strength enough in her arms to make up for the departed legs. Now we could move her from car to wheelchair and into the shops. Sometimes we would laugh together at our new way of doing things, yet sometimes we both knew we were laughing to keep from crying. Then one of us would say it again for her sake: "In some ways this really is the most fun we've ever had, don't you think?" Yet each of us knew that wasn't true.

We did share some great talks, though, really great talks, along these mountain roads. Almost every subject came up for discussion, including a new one for us. "Let's talk about heaven."

"Let's," I'd say, and wait for her to begin.

"Exactly what do you think Jesus meant when He said, 'In heaven we are neither married nor given in marriage?' I'm not sure I like that, Charlie. Do you suppose He meant it for a certain time and certain people? He couldn't have meant it for us, could He? Forty-eight years of love. The Lord I know wouldn't do that to us."

And I would answer, "The Lord I know wouldn't do that to us either."

Then on to this conclusion. I quote exactly. I've heard it many times, and it will forever be one of my favorites:

> "Don't you worry, Charlie. If I get to heaven before you do, I promise. If they're still operating on this 'no marriage' thing I'll have some special sessions with the Lord. I can almost guarantee He'll give us permission to be live-in buddies for all eternity."

Then we would shift to other subjects, but some of them still related to heaven.

All our lives Martha and I had lived with a weighty problem. My weight, never hers. She had one of those always-exactly-right bodies. Every day she tipped the scales where the needle should be.

Yet svelte as she was, she was almost always gracious about my proclivity to put on pounds. I say "almost" because it took some time for her to learn that all us fatties are alike. Losing weight is an inside job, inside the fatty. But whenever I did want to shape up from the inside out, she would approach it seriously. Queen of the culinary arts, she would be queen of the dietary dishes too. Cooking for me, eating with me, thrilling with me over my losses. Every sign that I was coming to contours more like the Lord's original made us both glad.

All this leads to another favorite Martha-musing from our heaven talk:

> "I used to wonder," she would begin, "about all the people in heaven. Think of it—billions of people from way back forever and ever. But don't worry, I can find *you*, Charlie. You'll be at the heavenly smorgasbord, pigging out on creamy desserts."

Then she would laugh, and I would too. So like Martha. Even in the darkness there must be something around here good for a smile. Maybe we could even manage a laugh.

But in these heavenly talk times we would discuss serious things too. Would she know her sister in heaven, the one who died in infancy? Would she be grown up now or still a baby? Could she be both grown up and small, depending on the time or the occasion? These questions too we would discuss and discuss again. As the poet says, "Ever we came out the same door we went in." But not always; sometimes we both knew we had been in touch with the Lord in these long talks. And isn't it good, so good, to reach eternal truth with one's best friend?

My best friend, Martha, was so childlike in her faith, yet so profound. Sometimes when she made a statement, I thought,

"She must have gone sixty fathoms deep for *that* one." But she also had the ability to make her deepest findings clear.
How?

> I think I have the answer here:
> Martha knew the Lord intimately.
> So many ways she knew Him:
> Creator, Redeemer,
> Guide, Inspiration.
> But more than any of these
> He was her Inner Presence,
> her personal friend
> for all eternity.

Bless thou the gifts our hands have brought,
Bless thou the work our hearts have planned.
Ours is the faith, the will, the thought;
The rest, O God, is in thy hand.

Longfellow

The Table Spread

One of our friends says that my idea of heaven is "significantly deficient in maturity." Does he mean "childish"? I hope he means "childlike." Didn't Jesus say, "Except ye become as little children, ye shall not enter the kingdom of heaven"?

What will heaven be like? The Bible gives very few clues. Did the Lord do this deliberately? Was He leaving empty spaces so we could fill in the gaps with our imagination?

Are there assignments for nurses in heaven? Yes, yes. Karen proved that to us all. There must be other special assignments, then, perhaps assignments for the culinary experts too.

Cookies, cakes, custards, and casseroles, dishes of infinite variety. Some still warm, some to be warmed, and even the cold offerings warm with the bearer's love.

So welcome. These are the days when I shiver in my soul and I need warming. If you are a taker of food to the needy (the needy of heart), I thank you.

To write of Martha's impending death and not include our family would never do. Peter, our professor son, coming with his big hug and, "How you doing, Dad?" Margie too, he brought, and is she ever the bringer of food! Our three other sons, Philip in Houston, Paul in San Francisco, and Timothy in New York, couldn't be with us except in mind and soul.

(But that's another great gift of God, isn't it? "Present in mind and soul.")

How did they do it, Peter and Margie? Together, they're church school teachers. He's a writer of books on real estate law. She's a president of our city Junior League. They are parents of two small children.

Yet here they came, night after night, spreading a banquet on our table. Our dishes, their food. Nine of us, gathered for a family sacrament. Karen and her daughters, busy, busy university students, there to care. All of us sharing, laughing (again, to keep from crying), waiting.

Could the Lord ever have done anything finer than placing us together in families? Then, as a bonus, providing friends for our extended family?

Thank you, thank you, Lord.

═══════

"You Need a Hand to Hold and a Face to Look At"

Karen and her mother had always been good friends. (Well, maybe some exceptions in junior high.) Now during the cancer days, daughter-nurse, mother-patient became woman-to-woman friends.

Sometimes when the moment was exactly right, Karen would ask, "Mama, are you afraid to die?"

"No. No," Martha would answer, "I'm not afraid to die. But I'd like to live, to live out my life with your daddy, loving him to the very end."

From here, I don't know everything Martha said, but I suppose it was some of the same she said to me: "I'd like to see my grandchildren grown, all those beautiful girls—Kristy, Martha Marie, Misty, Windy, Amanda, and now little Anna—each one so special. What will they become? Kristy might be our politician, and Martha, the veterinarian. Who will be the nurse? The doctor? Who will they marry? I'd like to know! How many children will they have? I'd like to know that too, because then I'd be a great-grandmother. How many times a great-grandmother, do you suppose?

"And Jarrett [her only grandson]. He's exhibit A of all the grandsons, isn't he? His daddy says Jarrett's middle name should be Search-and-Destroy, but he's such a good little boy for three, really. What do you think he'll be? Something great. Yes, I'd like to live, but afraid to die? No. No. I'm not afraid to die. What I am afraid of is leaving Charlie."

———

They must have had this discussion often, because Karen would tell me about it. Then I'd know that another conversation would follow soon, this one between Martha and me.

"Charlie, I want to talk with you about what you'll do if I die" (never "when," always "if").

"If I die, will you remember I reminded you the Bible has hardly begun until it says, 'It is not good for man to live alone'? That's your verse, Charlie. Who will cook for you? Who will write your checks and balance your checkbook? Who will keep up with your insurance and pay your taxes? "That's not all, who will share your deepest thoughts? Who will laugh with you, take trips with you? All that love you have in your heart, all the things you've learned loving me, who will share these with you? Will you remember sometimes that I said this? 'You need a hand to hold and a face to look at.' "

I will bring down the curtain on other things in these conversations. Some memories are just for the two of us: types, characteristics, personalities, histories, what to look for, what not to get involved in, all these she talked about. Classified conversations, though, meant only for Charlie and Martha.

Except:

I would like you to know she told me this: "If I die, I promise, when I get to heaven, the Lord and I will be thinking of you. And we'll both be so happy when you find someone to love and be loved by again."

Could there ever be any more beautiful gift from a wife who wanted to live but knew she wouldn't?

The gift of freedom . . .
    freedom from life's overzealous regulators of behavior,
    freedom to think for oneself,
    freedom of timing,
    freedom from guilt,
    freedom to hear clearly what the Lord says personally.

How many times have I felt these "if I die" blessings in my soul? And how many times have I praised the Lord for a dying wife who would say to her living husband:

> "You need a hand to hold
> and a face to look at."

Ask the very beasts,
and they will teach you;
ask the wild birds—
they will tell you,
This the Eternal's way.

Job 12:7, Moffatt

Kinship with All Life

Manx cats are not your ordinary, pedestrian cats. In the official nomenclature we call them "Stumpies" (short tail) and "Rumpies" (no tail). The back legs of Manx cats make them high behind, and they are leapers to great heights. If there were derbies for cats, it would be no contest. Without a tail holding them back, Manx cats are very, very fast. When they turn it up to high and hop like a kangaroo, they can outrun almost anything. But there are other differences more important.

The well-bred Manx has an altogether different philosophy from even its fancy cousins. And this is the difference. Cat fanciers know that most cats will rub against whatever leg is available for one reason only. It makes the cat feel good! But Manx cats, somewhere in their evolving, turned a corner. From then on life for them was not first to be loved but to love! Henceforth they would rub against people's legs to make the *people* feel good!

And that brings us to Dinah. Dinah is our current family cat, and how we got her is a story in itself. Early in our marriage Martha and I had raised Manx cats as a hobby. (That's how I know what I know about Manx cats.) So in our retirement, we decided to look for a Manx; a nice memento of the happy cat years. But no luck. No Manx.

Our next favorite cat being calico, we decided to settle for second choice. We studied the classified ads, and one night here it was.

> Found. Calico kitten. Very gentle female. If she be-longs to you, won't you please call 749–2738.

She wasn't ours—not then—but taking a chance, we di-aled the number to leave our name. "In case the true owners don't surface, please put us on your interested list."

"What list?" they asked. "You're the first to call. Can't you come right away? We're allergic to cats. Please. We've run the ad for two weeks without one single call. Please come and look at her. Please."

So I went, alone. Martha wasn't feeling well, which was very unusual. Looking back now, I know these must have been the first days of her last days.

When I arrived at their door, the whole family came to meet me: father, mother, daughter, son, two of them wheez-ing—and one small calico feline, purring.

But that's not all. What I tell you now I could hardly believe. This was a calico Manx! (A very rare combination, but typically Manx in every way, including one I forgot to mention: great greeters.)

They welcomed me in and immediately began to explain, "She doesn't have a tail, but we can almost guarantee you'll love her anyway."

And we did. Martha took to the little lady immedi-ately, and the little lady to Martha. It was love at first sight both ways.

"Only you must understand, little lady," Martha said, "all cats in our family are outdoor cats." Martha's rule, an established rule from day one with our first cat.

We named her Dinah. All our Manx cats had biblical names—Phinehas, Artaxerxes, Saul, Keturah, Dorcas, Mehetabel, and Mary (born on Christmas day). And now, Dinah, from the story of Leah, who bore her husband son after son after son, up to six. And then came this tender addition: "Later she bore a daughter whom she named Dinah" (Gen. 30:21).

Dinah did not like Martha's "No cats in the house" rule, for weeks she would slip in at every opportunity. And she was a genius at hiding when we went to catch her. Since Martha couldn't abide cats in the house, I really worked at this. "Dinah, rules being what they are, you are turning out to be pure nuisance. Slip in, hide, be seized, out you go—this has to end. The energy level isn't up to it any longer, Dinah. My attention from this day on cannot be given to chasing cats. Please try to understand."

Do you believe cats can comprehend human emergencies? Is it possible for them to finally get a message which calls forth sympathy? I believe that's possible. I know it was with Dinah. I tell you true; from that day on it was almost pathetic. Days, weeks, the little calico cat sat outside our den door. Looking in, she seemed to be asking, "Won't somebody come out to hold me, pet me, visit?"

Why had she stopped dashing for the interior whenever the door opened? Why this patient waiting now?

Then one night weeks later, Martha had a sinking spell, way down. This was the beginning of the scary times. Down, down to the border, but then she'd come back, and we would hope again. Sometimes we would be hopeful together. Sometimes when she'd go too far away, I would be hopeful alone.

It was one of those "so alone" days when Dinah broke the rule. Now, when the den door opened, completely out of character for her these days, here she came. Mad dash through the door, mad dash for Martha's room, up on Martha's bed, settle down, way down, purr from way down.

Is there any sound more soothing than the rhythmic purring of a cat? Probably only one thing more soothing, and that is the purr of a loving cat, like Dinah.

I will never forget that moment, a moment of holy meaning. As I sat there beside them, slowly Martha came back, back to consciousness. She opened her eyes, looked around, saw who her visitor was, and said, "Kitty?!" Question mark? Exclamation point! Next she turned to me and smiled her "This is so fine" smile. Then she fell away again. From that point on Dinah stayed in Martha's bed or on her lap. Only now and then she took brief leave to come and check on me.

=====

"Kinship with all life" is a provocative term. It is used frequently by experts who have majored in animal-human relationships. The term means different things to different people, some rather far out. But it certainly isn't too far out to believe that the Book of Genesis is right when it says, "God made them all, and He was pleased."

Did He make all life for an interlocking support system? If He did, shouldn't the entire system be treated with care by all for the sake of all? The serious observer cannot but respect every aspect of God's creation: the earth, the air, people, animals, plants, and all growing things. If God created them all, then we must respect them all, for all of them interlock. Don't they?

⎯⎯⎯⎯

Why were we, former breeders of Manx cats, lovers of Manx cats, looking for a Manx cat in this town? Why right now did some unknown family lose their calico kitten? Why did she make her way to a home where there were allergies to cats? Why did her original owners fail to look at "Lost and Found" in the classified ads? Why did Dinah sit patiently outside the door when she finally understood the house rules? And why did she, that particular way-down day, bound through the door to dash for a bed where she could bring her blessing?

That smile Martha smiled when Dinah came to her bed said more to me than I have told you. "No cats inside" was Martha's rule, not mine. This was never a point of contention between us. We saved our contention for bigger things (well, not always, but we tried)!

So this was one of these items understood: "people in, cats out." Yet now when she smiled this particular moment out of her shadows, I knew the meaning of her smile. "Since we both believe in 'kinship with all life,' let her stay. I like her here."

It was another of the traits I appreciated in Martha. Stand your ground if it's one of those all-important laws never to be broken. But then again, time changes things and so do situations.

In this revision of the rules, then, Dinah served. Day after day, night after night, week after week she came faithfully. Dear little calico hospice lady, she came to purr, to comfort, to bless.

No question about it in my mind. I think Dinah too understood that when God created us, He decided this would be a good thing:

"Kinship with all life!"

From Pure Joy springs all creation,
By Joy it is sustained,
Toward Joy it proceeds
And to Joy it returns.

Sanskrit saying

———————

Sending Her Valuables on Ahead

She was going on a long trip soon, and she knew it. She didn't know when, but she did know where. She also knew another thing: where she was going she would have a new body.

Cancer is an utter degradation for some. When the spinal cord is affected and legs no longer support, when hearing is impaired and even the voices of love are dim, when shades are drawn over the eyes and sight will not come clear—isn't this enough, Lord?

"Are the lilies still blooming by the fence, Charlie?
And the red azaleas at the porch, tell me about them."
This was Martha asking my eyes to see for her.

Awesome, agonizing, awful, all these and more. Then the functions go, the final degradation.

Final? Not quite. Slowly the mind begins to go too. This is the last of her valuables, and she's sending them all ahead.

How do I know? Her cascade of questions, same questions over and over. It's as though what thoughts she does have are clamoring for clarity.

Every day I lift her from her bed. I put her frail body in the wheelchair. I move her to the gliding rocker, the one at our bay window. No, she cannot see the dogwood, the redbud. The trees, so proud, shaping up to celebrate the spring, these too she cannot see. Does all this hurt her? Me, it hurts with a dreadful hurt. I hope she cannot hurt as I hurt.

Then my whole world comes tumbling in around me. This is the final hurt, the crushing query: "Do I know you? Who are you?"

Desolation . . . and the requiem of a broken heart:

"This has to be the final degradation, Lord.
I feel so utterly destroyed.
Nothing left with which to know me.
This can't go on. This has to end.
Please take her."

Now I have told Him, and I sit here stunned, forever stunned. Those who have been here tell me it is forever. Forever I will carry this guilt. "Take her, Lord. Yes, take her."

Now it is time to feed her—the morning bran, her fruit, a sip of coffee. I watch her. I love her. She doesn't know me. Everything is gone now; nothing left to commune with me, nothing left to commune with the Lord.

Then in the quiet, the awful quiet, I hear a voice. Isn't this the voice of a heavenly angel come to set me straight?

"Why are you so earthbound? Why so presumptuous?
When everything else is gone, doesn't the soul have
eyes to see the Lord? Doesn't it have a voice to talk
with Him and a hand to reach out and touch His hand?
Don't you remember He said, 'I will *never* leave you
nor forsake you!' "

I do remember. So now, breakfast done, I sit here
longer and muse. My thought clears.

I *had* forgotten He said that,
and in the darkness
I am grateful.

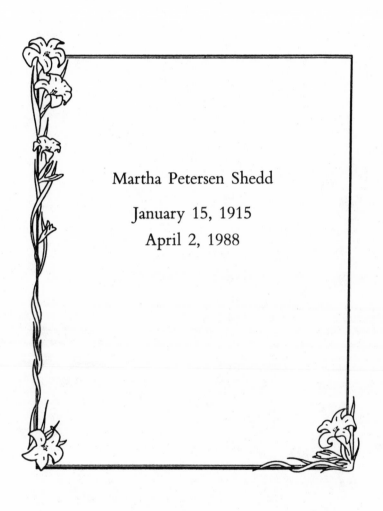

Martha Petersen Shedd

January 15, 1915

April 2, 1988

BROKEN PIECES

> You do not realize now what I am
> doing, but later you will understand.
>
> *John 13:7, NIV*

═══════

Easter Morning and I Am Angry

Each year as spring came, Martha and I seemed to stand on tiptoe waiting for Easter. With new life bursting all around, we felt a new sense of the Risen Presence. Especially we felt it inside.

Nearly always our Easter Day began with sunrise service. Then home for breakfast and Martha's culinary expertise at its epitome. After that off to church, filled with worshipers, overflowing. Services as they should be every Sunday. Celebrate, people, celebrate! Sing, choir, sing! Play, organ, play! Preach, preacher, preach! Christ the Lord is risen today!

Worship ended, see the long line, the greeting line, greeting each other, greeting the pastor. See the new clothes, new hats, new faces, or were some of them only looking new because they've been so long away? But never mind. "Happy Easter." "Happy Easter to you."

═══════

Now Martha is gone. Death is so insensitive. All these agonizing months and then the day before Easter? All right, all right, I'll be at the sunrise service, but will there be any sun? All this darkness in my soul. No sun.

It is very early Easter morning, and I am sitting on the love seat waiting for Karen. She will be down any time now, and we'll go together. Sunrise service on the steps of our church, up, up off the highway on a hill. The church seems even higher this year with the lofty new steeple. All freshly painted white. White as in pure white. White as in mausoleum white. We will be there, Karen and I. We will listen, be reverent, cry, leave early.

Suddenly, while I sit here on the love seat waiting, comes a rushing flood of anger. On our love seat? Wrong setting for anger, but here it comes. Fierce, frightening—thrilling too in its honesty, cleansing in its aftermath.

For me, my talk with the Lord that Easter morning will forever be a mighty episode of brutal exchange between friends. Here we are, friends shouting to be heard. This is a new dimension of rage and—soothing, ugly, scary—a new way to pray. "Horrors! What am I saying? What am I doing?"

"Lord," I begin, "you listen up. I'm angry with you. You did us wrong. You let us down. You messed up the script. I hope you're ashamed. From that terrible day in August, that day they found her cancer, don't you remember? From that day we've been praying for a miracle, a miracle by Easter. Plenty of time for you, plenty of time to stop this yo-yo. A touch of good news, and up we'd go. 'Oh, thank you, Lord, for hearing our prayers.' A glimmer of hope, a wave of gratitude, and, give us credit, we *never* forgot to thank you. Then bad news, bad signs, and down we'd go.

"So this is Easter and Martha is in heaven! And *that* is your miracle? Of course it's a miracle, but it's not the miracle we prayed for, and you know it. You want the truth? Here it is:

today, this Easter Day, I am angry. I do not even like you!"

Inside I shivered and shook. I also felt better. Much, much better, relieved. Then I waited. I listened. And now, clear as I ever heard God, these words came through, calm, understanding, almost as though He were suffering too:

> "Charlie, I know you don't like me today. That's all right. For me, it's no new thing. You didn't invent that. So many people haven't liked me—good people. Remember? Jesus didn't like me on the cross. 'Where have you been?' He said, 'Why have you forsaken me?' Read it again; you'll see. Moses didn't like me, and Abraham. Job didn't like me, and David, not even a little bit. Way back to Adam, I've heard it, 'Today I do not like you.' So understand me now, Charlie. I'm not asking you to like me. I'm only asking that you love me."

"What else can I say? Forty-eight years with Martha, Lord, and the dogwood is blooming. How can I explain all these years with one of your angels and the dogwood too? How can I explain so many things unless I love you? All right, I'll love you, but I don't like you."

Then the closure. "Good," He said. "If you will love me, some day in your future I will show you wonders you couldn't imagine now. Wonders for Martha. Wonders for you."

"Well," I answered, "it better be good for Martha now."

"It is," He said, "and it will be for you. This is how it's always been. If you go on loving me, never stop loving me, I promise, here, hereafter, you will like me again."

Now, it is two years later, two years with that whole new dimension in my prayer life. Total honesty between the Lord and me. Today I am beginning to see what He meant.

Most of the time I do like Him again, and I can believe again.

I believe that as certainly as the
   oak is hidden within the acorn,
as sure as the rose lies deep
   in the bud,
so too in our hearts is stamped
   the ultimate plan of God,
the loving plan of a loving heavenly Father,
   who, though He seems to be long gone,
is always there,
   molding, shaping, reshaping,
using even the night of our crucifixion
   to bring a resurrection in the morning,
     if we let Him.

Weeping may endure for a night, but joy
cometh in the morning.

Making Shore on Broken Pieces

It must have been a terrible shipwreck. The Apostle Paul
was on his way to Rome. He had advised the captain against
putting out to sea, but his warning went unheeded. They
sailed, and when the winds came, everyone knew they were
in for big trouble.

Rocking and reeling, even the sailors began to panic.
"What can we do?" Superstitious as they were, they could
begin with the old familiar question: "Has anyone on board
made the gods angry?"

Then came the shipwreck. Too late for mumbo jumbo, the
ship is driven into a shoal. Grounded. Now all these fierce
winds, all these high waves beating on the stern are too much.
This ship is done. "See it bend. Feel it break. Swim, men, swim
for shore!"

What about the nonswimmers, the weak, those so terrified
they have forgotten how to swim? "Do not worry," says Paul,
"we all made it to shore, some on boards and some on broken
pieces of the ship."

All? Two hundred sixty-six were on board. All made it?
Unbelievable, yes, plus encouraging. Especially encouraging
to me.

During some of the low times in her closing days, Martha
and I had shared this story together. Now, at her death, our

ship broken in two, I seemed drawn back to Acts 27 and Paul's shipwreck.

Interesting how some Scripture passages insist that we read and reread, study and restudy. Only when we have served our time in them do they give up their personal message. This one finally did for me. The personal message came clear, no more questions: "You must not quit, Charlie. Hold fast to your board. Paddle on. Two hundred sixty-six made it from Paul's ship. Millions and millions have made it since the beginning of time. You *can* do it."

How?

Pondering, planning, praying, I came up with certain helps and warnings which were like life preservers in the choppy sea. I call them my affirmations for making shore on broken pieces.

1.   *I Refuse to Drown in Self-Pity.*

"Behold and see if there be any sorrow like unto my sorrow." Of course there is. Am I the most pitiful of all these clinging to boards and broken pieces? I doubt it.

My requiem of woe does not do me well out here. It saps my energy. It isolates me in a miserable whirlpool of selfishness. Say it again, stronger this time: "I refuse to drown in self-pity."

2.   *I Will Not Talk Too Much.*

Crazy people say crazy things. They do crazy things too, and I am crazy now. Simply understanding that I am somewhat insane with grief sets up important guards to both my words and my actions.

If I accept myself as I am, temporarily off balance and abnormal, I have done a good thing for myself and for others around me. I must keep a filter on my lips and a firm hand on my behavior.

3.   *I Will Get Help From the Right People.*

The right people may come singly or in groups. Because there are so many who have suffered as I suffer, I can find support if I remain open to it: churches, fellowships, professionals, seminars, workshops, amateurs, friends.

If I look for them, I will find those who understand. Somewhere I can surface my bewilderment, but not to everyone. Part of this lonesome valley I must walk by myself, but not all of it.

4.   *I Will Do Something for Others.*

We have a lot of company out here in these choppy waters. So paddle this broken piece of ship over to some fellow struggler. It will help me in my struggle. Is there any man who has had life exactly the way he wanted it? Any woman? Any child?

When I open my ears to the SOS calls around me, I hear
parents agonizing over their children;
> children agonizing "Why is my father too busy
> for me?" "Why is my mother so sad?";
businessmen whose ships have gone down in
> economic storms;
the betrayed, who put their trust in someone not
> worthy of trust;
the divorced, crying at night, drowning in tears;
> Their waters of rejection must be even colder
> than my cold waters.

the sick, tired, despairing, the catastrophe victims of
every kind.

Call the roll. They're all here. These, my fellows in the
tragedies of life, need from me a touch of the hand, a lift, an
encouraging word.

Help me to remember too, Lord, that when I minister to
someone for you, you minister to me.

5.   I Will Get Ready Ahead of Time.

For some reason I had never once considered the possibility
that Martha might die first. Never a flickering thought in all
our years, and that's plain foolish. Without getting morbid,
remember, it is a fact, a somber fact, but true: "I may be the
leftover." The wise will consider this possibility ahead of time.

It *is* possible to prepare ourselves for the rough seas and
storms that wreck our boats. When our ship begins to come
apart, we may not have time to run for the life preservers.
Before we know it, here we are in the cold, cold water. Now
whether we make it may depend on what we've been doing
before the ship broke up.

The practice of daily prayer year after year after year, an
ongoing program of personal Bible study, faithful worship—
all these strengthen the soul for calamities we could not see
when skies were blue.

As she was dying, Martha and I turned often to our
favorite scriptures. Here we found verses, passages, whole
books of the Bible calling for our new attention. And that was
a very good thing too. Some passages lie dormant until the day
of need.

In that category for us was the superb Old Testament book
of Lamentations. Why had we hurried through it before?

Perhaps it was because the very name seems to say, "It will be sad in here."

One day as we were reading, some of the verses began breaking apart. Phrases, meanings, groups of words bound themselves together in a litany. This was Lamentations speaking just to us, ministering to us. Then, as if in a whisper meant only for me, I thought I heard, "Write these words on your heart. One day they may minister to you alone."

And they did.

A Litany for Those Who Suffer

How solitary and lonely sits the city. . . . Behold our sorrow and suffering. . . . Our sighs and groans are many. . . . Our emotions are deeply disturbed, and our eyes overflow with tears.

We are walled about, and we have been brought into darkness. . . . Perished is our strength, and our ruin seems measureless.

Yet because of the love of the Lord we are not consumed. . . . Great is His faithfulness. . . . He remains and reigns forever. . . . Therefore we hope in Him and expectantly wait.

(Verses from the Old Testament Book of Lamentations. Amplified Version, with adaptations. Selected and arranged by Charlie and Martha Shedd. February 1, 1988)

6. I Will Head for the Promised Shoreline.

This is the hope that keeps me afloat. Here, hereafter my
feet may stand again on solid ground. I will not succumb to
the assumption that all is lost in the blackness.

Black it is. And by itself black has little beauty. No con-
trast, nothing to blend with it. Dark, dank, dismal.

As I feel myself sinking in this blackness, I reach out for
another piece of help, of hope, and I am reminded of a story
Martha and I shared often. Especially we shared it as her dark
days darkened.

=====

One of my seminary professors had served as president of
our denomination's Board of World Mission. In this position
he traveled to many countries, which fit very well his number
one hobby. Being a connoisseur of art, he visited great mu-
seums everywhere.

His favorite art works were murals. He had seen the best.
He loved the old, but especially he said, "One of my greatest
thrills is to see a new mural unveiled."

One day while attending a conference in France he read
of an unveiling next day at the Louvre. It was one of those
masterful sea pieces covering an entire wall, a mural called *The
Shipwreck.* This one he must see!

Hurrying on down to the Louvre, where he knew the head
guard, he asked a special favor. Because he had to leave that
night for a meeting in Africa, could the guard accommodate
him for a private unveiling?

Not an unusual request, he said, but to it came an unusual
answer.

"I'm sorry, my friend," the guard replied, "I wish I could
do what you ask, but I can't. Our contract with this artist

forbids the unveiling of his mural until it is unveiled for all. However, because you are a special friend, I can afford you this slight favor. You may go to a corner and lift the curtain to view that much."

"So I went," the professor said. "But when I lifted the curtain there was only one color, black, the blackest of blacks. Of course, I turned to look at the guard, and he, understanding my thoughts, said, 'I know what you're thinking, but because we are friends you will believe me, won't you? I have seen the entire mural, and I can promise you the black blends with all the other colors to make the total mural beautiful.' "

Blessed are the sad who
hold on to the faith that God,
the Great Artist, is able
to blend this blackest of black
with all His other colors
to make life beautiful again.

Martha believed that
and I believe it too:
"Weeping may endure for a night,
but joy cometh
in the morning."

DEDICATION

It is a welcome change
when the hurting memories
begin to bless.
This book is dedicated
to the beautiful memories
of Martha.

"Remember, I love you too."

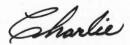

To contact Charlie Shedd regarding speaking engagements, write or call Michael McKinney, McKinney Associates, Inc., P.O. Box 5162, Louisville, KY 40205, (502) 583-8222.